THE NEW ATKINS DIET COOKBOOK

Your Comprehensive Guide to Achieving Optimal Health and Weight Loss Through Delicious and Easy-to-Follow Low-Carb and High-Protein Recipes

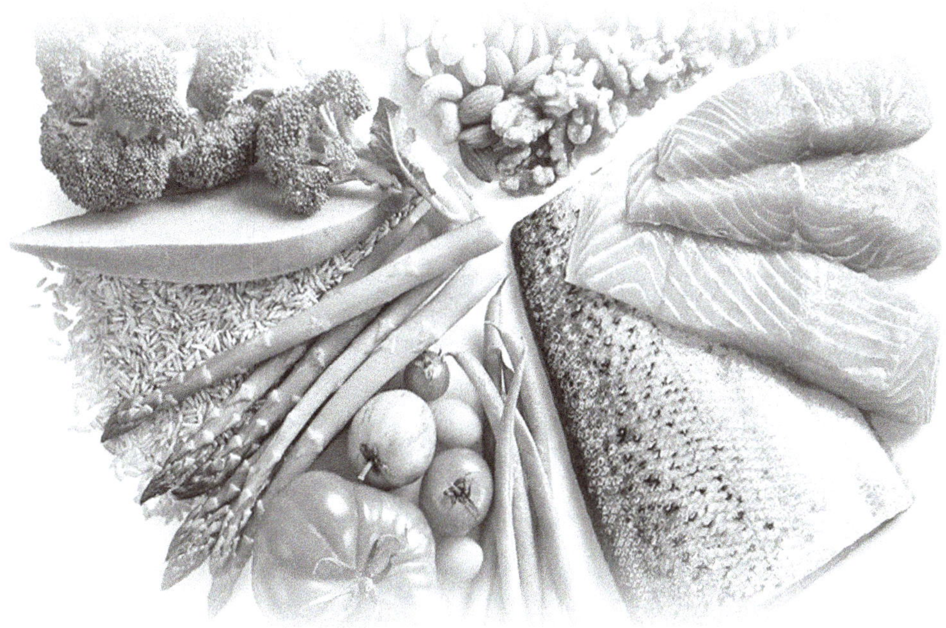

Dr. Sarah M. Patel

Copyright Statement and Disclaimer

Dear Reader,

Thank you for embarking on a culinary adventure through the pages of this recipe book. We appreciate your choice and enthusiasm for exploring the world of flavors presented herein. It is our joy to share our culinary passion with you, and we also want to provide clarity regarding the rights, responsibilities, and expectations associated with using this book.

Copyright Notice

Warm regards,

Dr. Sarah M. Patel (RD)

TABLE OF CONTENTS

Chapter One: Understanding the Atkins Diet

- Explanation of ketosis and how the diet works
- The four phases of the Atkins Diet
- Foods to enjoy and avoid

Chapter Two: Getting Started

- Preparing your kitchen for the Atkins Diet
- Tips for dining out and handling social situations
- Incorporating exercise into your routine

Chapter Three: Breakfast

Chapter Four: Lunch

Chapter Five: Dinner

Chapter Six: Snack

Chapter Seven: Dessert

Chapter Eight

- Four-Week Meal Plan
- Grocery Shopping List
- Strategies for staying motivated on the Atkins diet
- Dealing with Plateaus

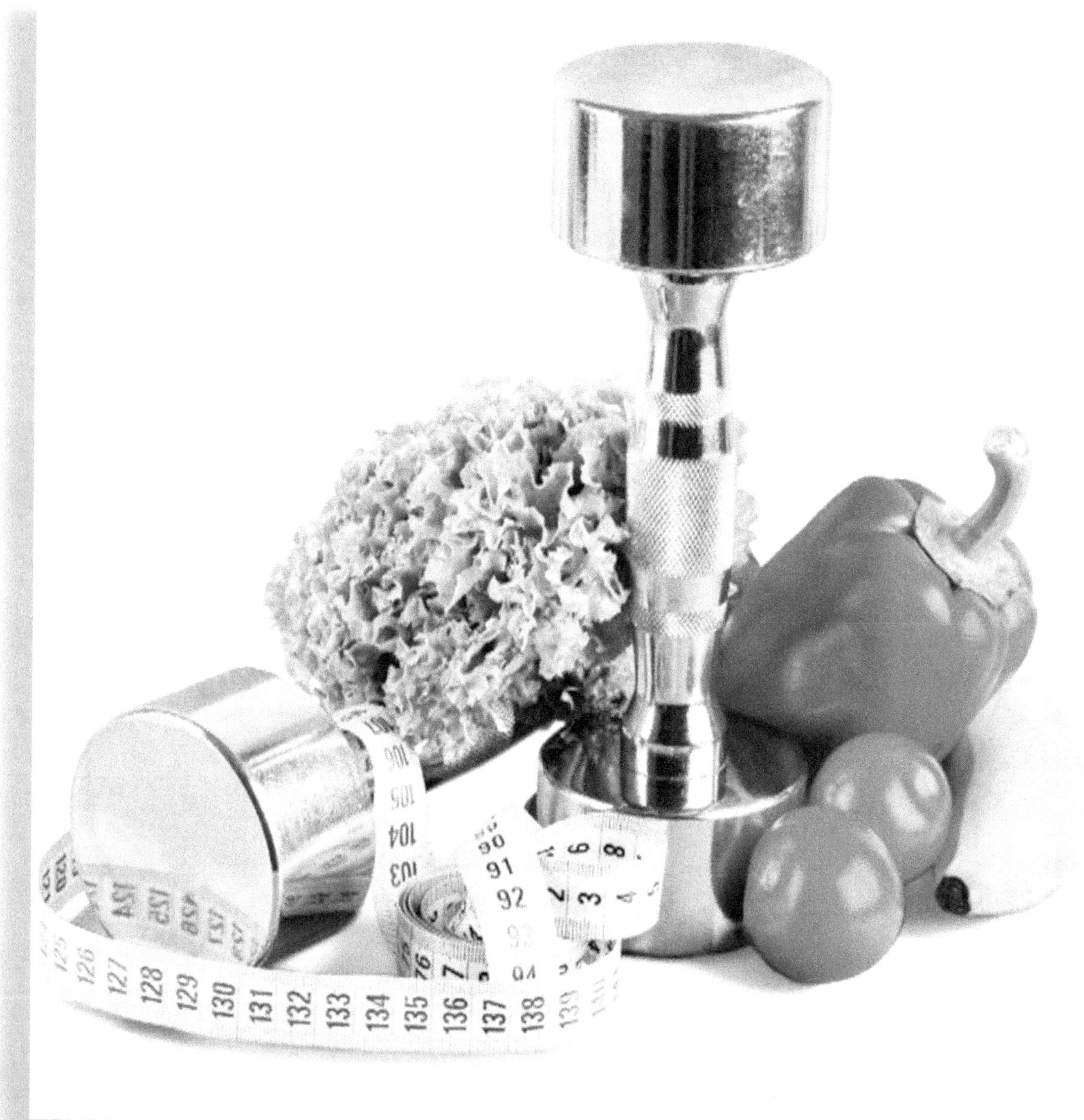

Introduction

Amidst the myriad of passing diet fads and fleeting wellness trends that inundate our world, the Atkins Diet emerges as a steadfast symbol of lasting success and scientific credibility. For decades, this revolutionary dietary approach has transformed lives, reshaping perceptions about weight loss, health, and vitality. As a seasoned professional in health and fitness, I am honored to introduce you to the definitive Atkins Diet Cookbook—a comprehensive compendium designed to empower you on your journey towards optimal health and well-being.

Founded by the visionary Dr. Robert C. Atkins in the early 1970s, the Atkins Diet revolutionized the way we perceive nutrition and weight management. At its core, the Atkins Diet is grounded in the fundamental principle of carbohydrate restriction to induce a metabolic state known as ketosis. By minimizing carbohydrate intake and prioritizing protein and healthy fats, this dietary approach triggers the body to burn stored fat for fuel, leading to rapid and sustainable weight loss.

The benefits of the Atkins Diet extend far beyond mere weight loss. Through meticulous research and clinical trials, the Atkins Diet has been scientifically proven to offer a myriad of health advantages, including improved blood sugar control, enhanced cardiovascular health, and heightened energy levels. By stabilizing blood sugar levels and reducing insulin resistance, the Atkins Diet can also be an effective tool in managing conditions such as type 2 diabetes and metabolic syndrome.

At the heart of the Atkins Diet lies a profound understanding of the body's metabolic processes and nutritional requirements. By embracing a low-carbohydrate, high-protein approach, individuals can recalibrate their metabolism, optimize fat-burning potential, and unlock newfound levels of vitality. Central to the Atkins philosophy is the concept of ketosis—a metabolic state wherein the body utilizes ketones derived from fat as its primary source of energy.

The Atkins Diet unfolds in four distinct phases, each meticulously designed to facilitate progressive weight loss and sustainable lifestyle changes. From the initial Induction phase, characterized by strict carbohydrate restriction, to the subsequent phases of Ongoing Weight Loss (OWL), Pre-Maintenance, and Maintenance, the Atkins Diet offers a structured roadmap towards achieving your health and wellness goals.

Navigating the dietary landscape can be daunting, but with the Atkins Diet, clarity reigns supreme. Embrace whole, nutrient-dense foods such as lean proteins, leafy greens, and healthy fats while minimizing or eliminating refined carbohydrates and sugars. By prioritizing real, wholesome ingredients, you'll nourish your body from the inside out, fueling it with the essential nutrients it craves for optimal performance and vitality.

Embarking on the Atkins Diet journey begins with a firm commitment to self-care and well-being. Prepare your kitchen for success by stocking up on Atkins-approved staples and purging your pantry of processed, carb-laden temptations. Arm yourself with strategies for dining out and navigating social situations with grace and confidence, ensuring that your commitment to health remains unwavering in any setting.

While diet plays a pivotal role in your journey towards optimal health, physical activity serves as its indispensable counterpart. Explore the myriad benefits of regular exercise, from bolstering metabolism and enhancing cardiovascular health to fostering a profound sense of well-being and vitality. Whether it's brisk walks, strength training, or yoga, find activities that resonate with your body and soul, and commit to making movement an integral part of your daily routine.

Embark on a culinary adventure with our meticulously crafted meal plans and tantalizing recipes. From hearty breakfasts and vibrant salads to sumptuous main courses and decadent desserts, our cookbook offers a diverse array of low-carb, high-protein dishes to tantalize your taste buds and nourish your body. Whether you're a novice in the kitchen or a seasoned chef, our recipes are designed to be approachable, delicious, and effortlessly aligned with the principles of the Atkins Diet.

As you journey towards optimal health and vitality, staying motivated and resilient is paramount. Learn how to navigate plateaus,

celebrate your successes, and gracefully transition from weight loss to weight maintenance. Armed with practical tips, shopping lists, and food diary templates, you'll have the tools and resources needed to embrace the Atkins lifestyle with confidence and conviction.

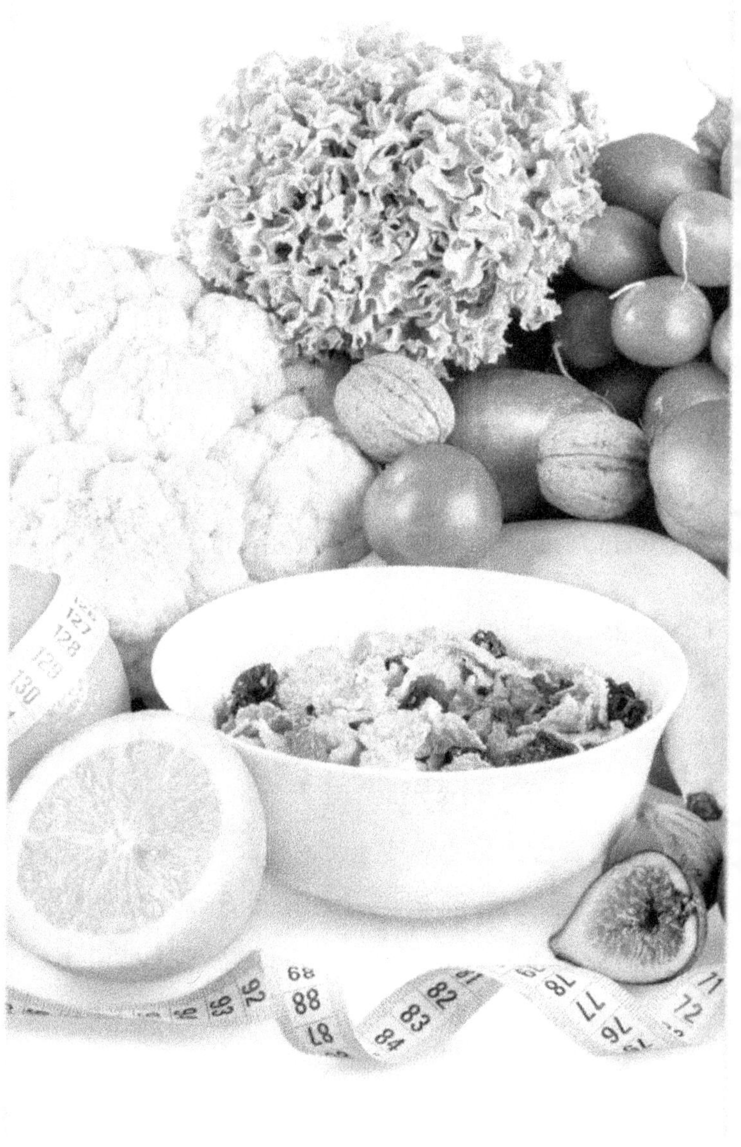

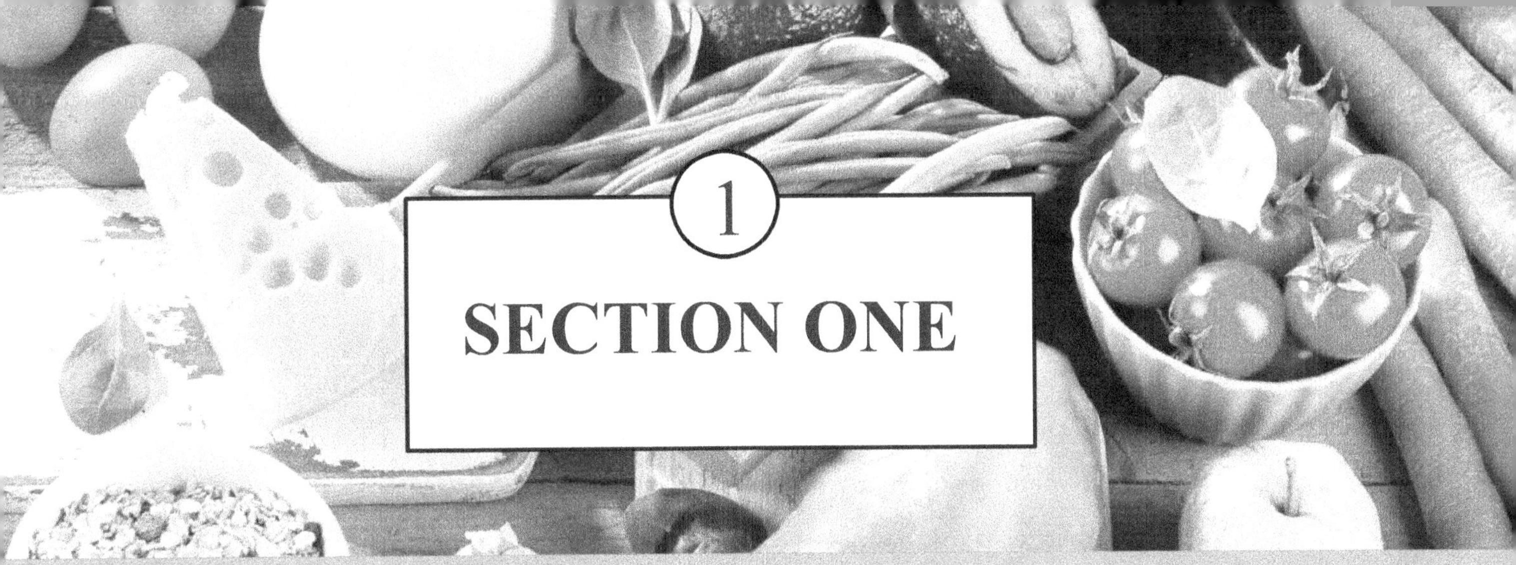

Ketosis and the Atkins Diet

The Atkins Diet is a low-carb, high-protein diet that stimulates your body's metabolism to burn fat more efficiently. This metabolic state is known as ketosis.

When you restrict your carbohydrate intake, your body starts to burn fat as fuel instead of glucose (sugar). This switch to burning fat releases ketones, which provide an alternate fuel source for the brain, have anti-inflammatory activities, and act as a mild appetite suppressant. This process of burning fat and producing ketones is what we call ketosis.

Ketosis is the most efficient path ever devised for getting you slim. The more ketones you release, the more fat you have dissolved. Lipolysis, the process of dissolving fat, is the biochemical method of weight loss. It's the alternative to using glucose for fuel, the very process that has made you heavy by storing excess glucose as fat.

The Atkins Diet leverages the process of ketosis to help you lose weight and maintain a healthy lifestyle. By understanding how ketosis works, you can use this knowledge to your advantage on your weight loss journey.

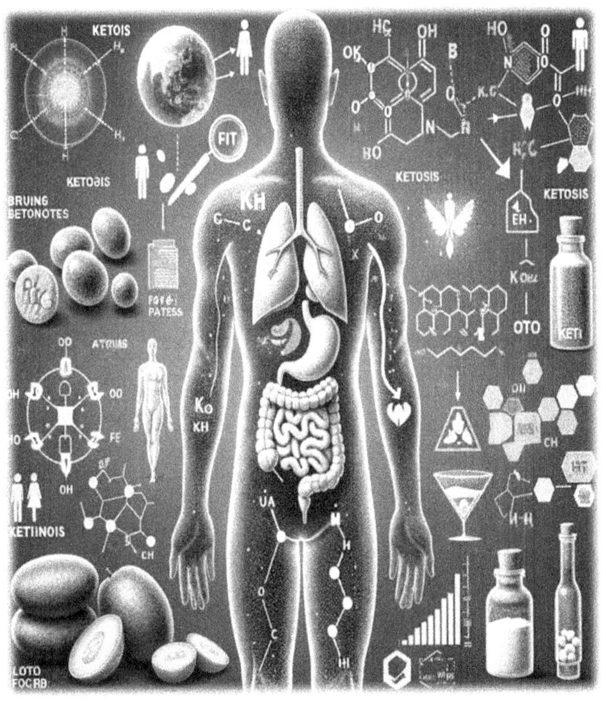

The Four Phases of the Atkins Diet

The Atkins Diet is divided into four phases:

Phase 1: Induction

The Induction phase is the first and strictest part of the Atkins Diet. In this phase, you consume under 20 grams of carbs per day for 2 weeks. The goal is to kick-start the weight loss by putting your body into a state of ketosis, where it burns fat for fuel instead of carbohydrates. During this phase, you eat high-fat, high-protein foods with low-carb vegetables like leafy greens.

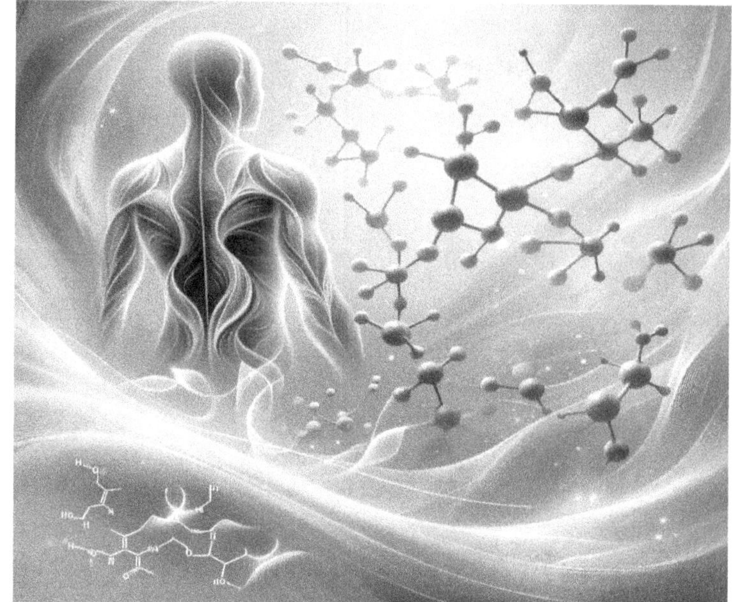

Phase 2: Ongoing Weight Loss (OWL)

In the OWL phase, you slowly add more nuts, low-carb vegetables, and small amounts of fruit back to your diet. You can consume between 25 and 50 net carbs daily. This phase lasts until you are about 10 pounds from your desired weight. The goal of this phase is to continue the weight loss at a slower, steadier pace.

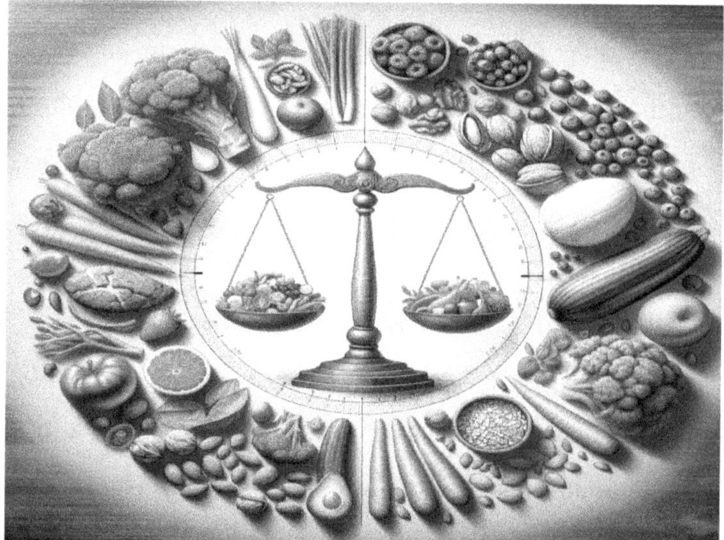

Phase 3: Pre-Maintenance

When you're very close to your goal weight, you add more carbs to your diet until weight loss slows down. You can consume 50 to 80 net carbs daily during this phase. The goal of the Pre-Maintenance phase is to find the maximum amount of carbs you can eat while not gaining or losing weight.

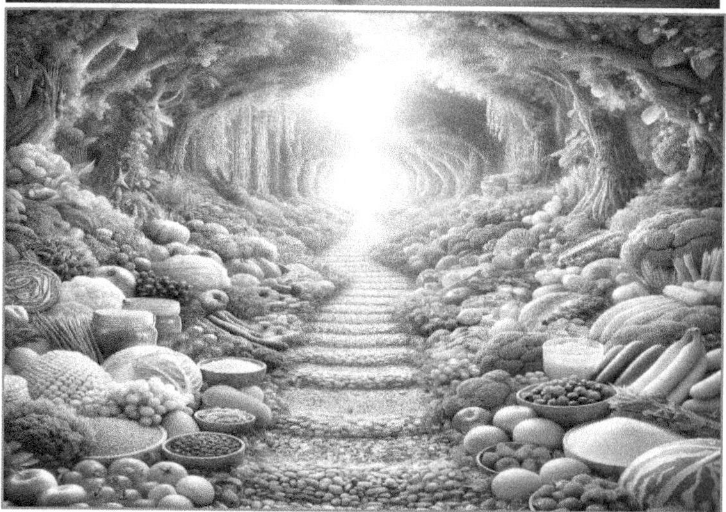

Phase 4: Lifetime Maintenance

Once you reach your ideal weight, you continue to eat a predominantly low-carbohydrate diet (80-100 net carbs per day) for life. The goal of the Lifetime Maintenance phase is to maintain your ideal weight and make the Atkins Diet a permanent lifestyle change.

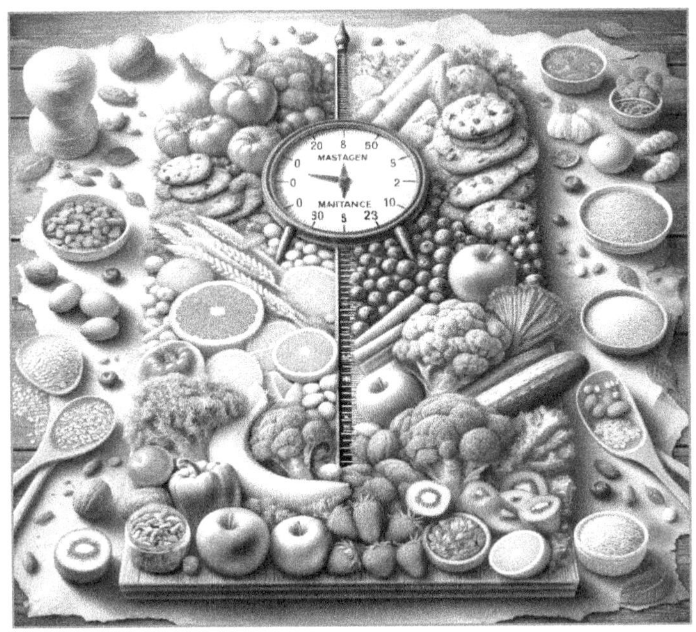

Foods to Enjoy and Avoid

The Atkins Diet encourages the consumption of a variety of foods, including meats, low-carb vegetables, and healthy fats. Here are some foods you can enjoy:

4. **Low-Carb Fruits:** Berries.

5. **Full-Fat Dairy:** Cheese and butter.

6. **Nuts and Seeds:** Almonds, walnuts, flaxseeds, chia seeds.

7. **Healthy Fats and Oils:** Olive oil, coconut oil, avocado oil.

1. **Meats:** Bacon, pork chops, lamb chops, chicken thighs, beef steaks, turkey slices, venison steaks.

2. **Fatty Fish and Seafood:** Sardines, mackerel, salmon, trout, tuna, herring, whitebait

3. **. Low-Carb Vegetables:** Spinach, broccoli, kale.

Foods to Avoid

Foods to avoid or limit, depending on the phase of the diet, here are some foods that you should avoid or limit while following the Atkins Diet:

3. **Starchy Vegetables:** Such as corn and potatoes.

4. **Fruits with High Sugar Content:** Such as pineapple, mango, papaya, and bananas.

1. **Sugary Foods:** Soft drinks, fruit juices, cakes, candy, ice cream, and similar products.

2. **Refined Grains:** Foods made with white flour or refined grains.

Remember, the types of foods to avoid or can vary depending on the phase of the diet you are in. It's always best to check the specific guidelines for each phase of the Atkins Diet.

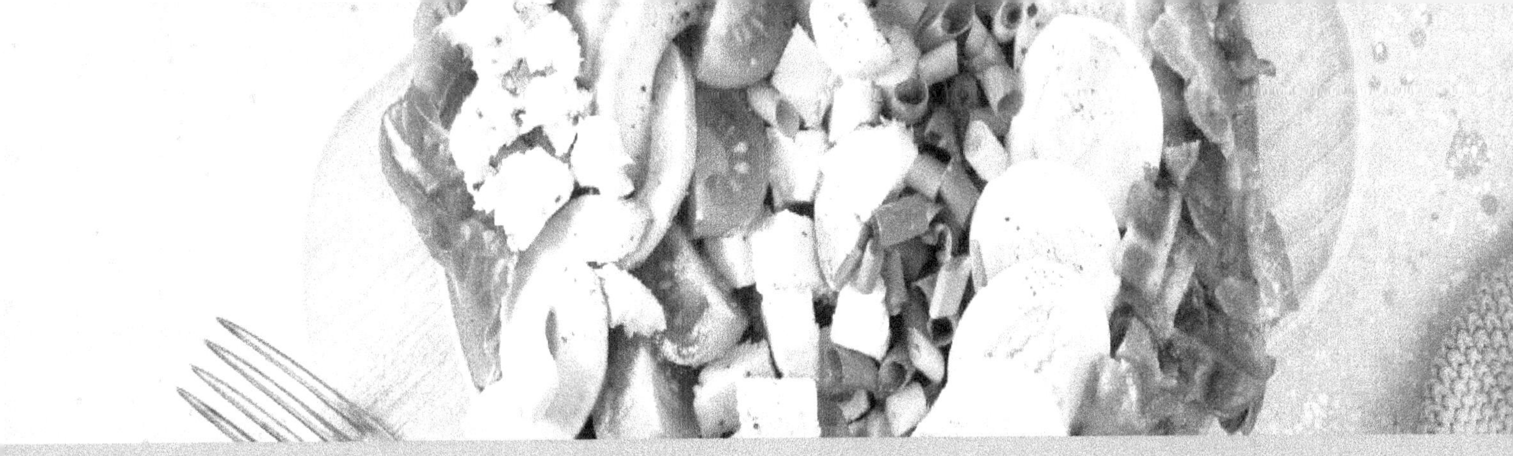

Preparing Your Kitchen for the Atkins Diet

Starting the Atkins Diet means shifting your nutritional focus to foods that are high in protein and healthy fats. Here are some detailed tips to prepare your kitchen:

Adjust Your Food Supply: Stock your pantry with Atkins-friendly foods. This includes unprocessed meat, poultry, seafood, eggs, low-carb vegetables, and healthy fats. You can also cook or grill up chicken, steak, and fish and portion and freeze. Defrost whenever you need your protein of choice for a meal during the week.

Plan Your Meals: Before you hit the grocery store, plan your meals and snacks for the week. Think about which ingredients you can use in multiple dishes. Use a carb counter to get a good idea of what foods you will add or eliminate from your diet.

Prep Your Veggies: Don't let fresh veggies languish in the refrigerator until they rot. Wash and cut them up and store them in clear glass containers as soon as you return from the store. That way you can grab them for snacks or quickly add them to omelets, main dishes, or salads.

Consider Canned Veggies: Fresh veggies are a great value for the price, but they can become costly if they spoil and you must throw them away. Augment your selection of fresh veggies with canned vegetables like tomatoes. They can be just as nutritious and cost-effective and are the perfect long-lasting pantry staples for many meals.

Use Grocery Apps: Many supermarkets have apps that offer discounts, coupons, and loyalty rewards. Stick to your list to prevent unnecessary spending. Have a low-carb snack before you go to the store to avoid hunger-induced impulse buys.

Repurpose Proteins: Roast a chicken (or buy a rotisserie chicken) for one meal and use leftovers for salads, wraps, or stir-fries. Add leftover steak or grilled chicken to a hearty salad for lunch or turn it into fajitas or tacos.

Batch Cooking: Also known as "cook once, eat twice." Start with one basic recipe that can be adapted into different dishes. Cook a large portion of meat sauce, like Bolognese, and portion into containers for your freezer to pull out when needed.

Remember, the goal is to stock your pantry with smart, delicious staples to keep your low-carb meals exciting, satisfying, and easy to prepare.

Tips for Dining Out and Handling Social Situations

Navigating social situations while on the Atkins Diet can be a challenge, but with a little preparation and knowledge, it's entirely possible. Here are some detailed tips:

Start with Salad: Vegetables are low in net carbs and packed with fiber, which means they are a great start to any meal. Always have a salad first, with as many greens as possible, before your main entrée, and you will avoid overdoing it.

Bring Your Own: Many people keep mini bottles of hot sauce or their favorite spices with them, and season their restaurant meals as needed when they eat out. When you go out to a restaurant, take your own dressing with you for your salad so that way you know exactly how many carbs you are getting.

Know Your Triggers and Avoid Them: Make a plan in advance on how you will avoid potential carb-filled pitfalls at your meal. Dining out is so easy on Atkins. By now you should know what you can have, and what a trigger food is. Don't feel bad asking to substitute the fries or potatoes with broccoli or Brussels sprouts.

Ask for a Substitute: Restaurants are in the service business. As long as you are polite to your server, he or she should be more than happy to accommodate most requests. When dining out, do not be afraid to ask to substitute items or have it made how you want it.

Master the Art of Fast Food: You may find yourself at the fast-food drive-thru more often than you like, thanks to busy work schedules, after-school sports, and more. It certainly is not a bad idea to cut down on your fast-food visits, but if you do go, there are options. For example, Wendy's has no problem making a double hamburger without a bun and letting you substitute a Caesar side salad for French fries.

Stay Hydrated and Have a Snack: Sometimes hunger can mimic thirst. So, it's important to stay hydrated and have a snack if you're feeling hungry.

Mindful Eating: Notice how good the food tastes, how hungry or satisfied you may be. Let your sensory experience, your chewing, and swallowing bring you back fully to eating. Keep your focus here for at least a few seconds. Then shift back to the social milieu. Focus on the conversation, mindfully listen, and contribute.

Avoid Food Table at Parties: Don't stand next to the food table at a party; the chances of you going back for seconds and thirds will be much higher.

Incorporating exercise into your routine

While exercise is not essential if you want to lose weight on the Atkins Diet, it does offer many benefits. Here are some detailed tips to incorporate exercise into your routine:

1. Understand the Benefits of Exercise: Exercise builds and maintains healthy muscles, bones, and joints, improves mood, boosts your energy, helps you maintain your weight loss, and helps prevent heart disease, diabetes, metabolic syndrome, and more. Regular exercise appears to reduce both depression and anxiety, improve mood and enhance the ability to perform daily tasks well into old age.

2. Start with a Basic Routine: If you're not yet working out, you can try a workout that combines high-intensity interval training (HIIT) and weight training. This workout can be done by anyone, in only 20 minutes a day.

3. Include Protein in Every Meal: The first thing your body needs for exercise is a fresh supply of amino acids from protein. Amino acids are the building blocks of protein and are used by your body for making muscles, hormones, neurotransmitters, bones, and all sorts of other important things. Exercise depletes critical amino acids like glutamine and the three branched-chain amino acids—valine, isoleucine, and leucine. When you eat protein, it replenishes your body's supply of these branched-chain amino acids. Think meat, chicken, eggs, fish, or whey protein.

4. Carbohydrates and Exercise: Exercise draws upon your body's stores of glycogen, which is the storage form of sugar.

Glycogen waits in your liver and your muscles for a signal that sugar is needed—kind of like "Hey, she's exercising, let's give her some fuel!". Your body can hold about 1,800 calories of sugar as glycogen, which is plenty to fuel any workout short of a marathon.

5. How Much Should You Exercise?: Most health organizations (such as the American College of Sports Medicine) have focused on endurance and have specified "sustained periods of vigorous physical activity involving large muscle groups and lasting at least 20 minutes on three or more days a week.". However, as research continues to accumulate, we now know that even small amounts of activity throughout the day will add up and produce benefits.

6. Weight Training: Your body burns calories and fat in tiny structures in the cell called the mitochondria, which are like Power Central for the cell. And mitochondria are found mainly in the muscle cells. Therefore, weight training needs to be added into the mix.

Notes:

Your
Observation:

Progress
Report:

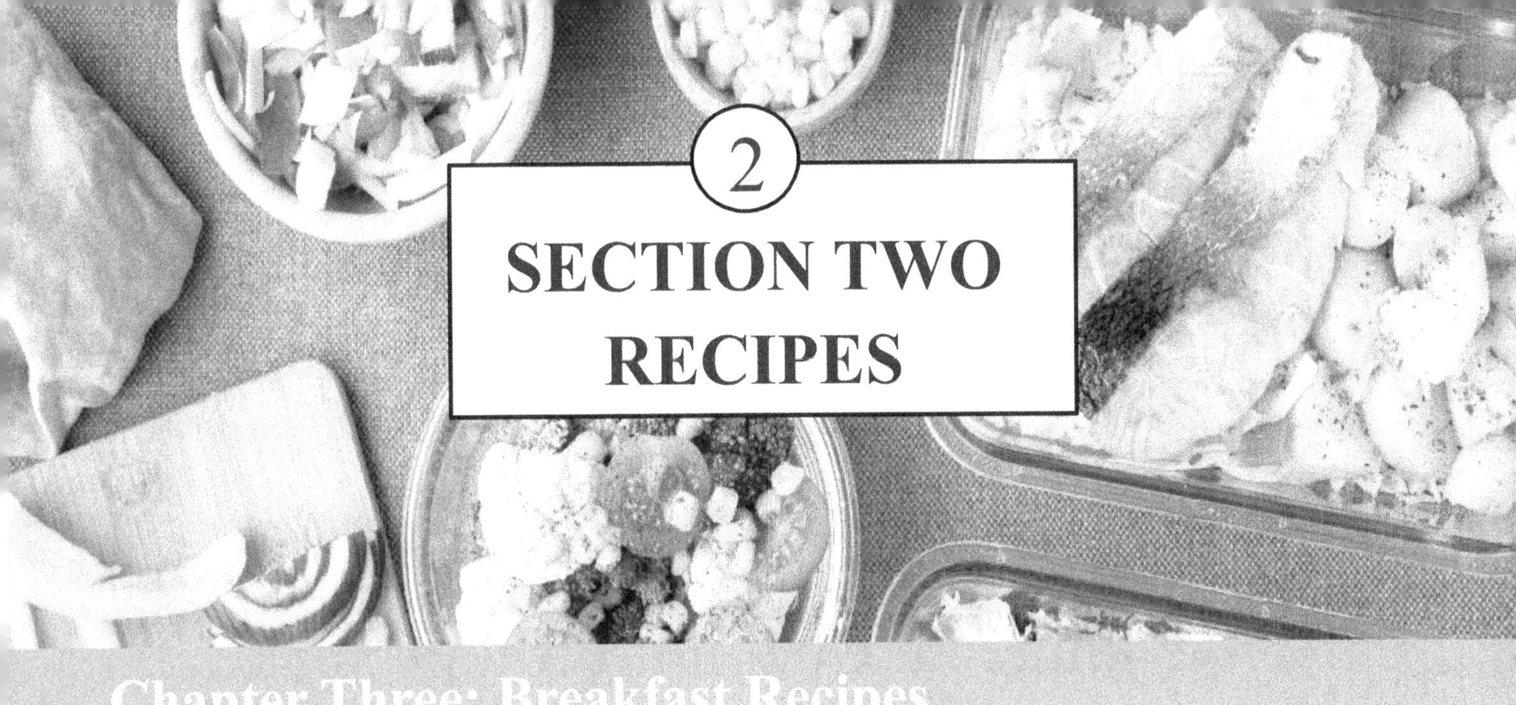

Keto Sausage Egg Cups

SERVINGS: 6   PREP TIME: 15 MINUTES   COOK TIME: 30 TO 50 MINUTES

- 6 eggs
- 1/2 cup cooked sausage
- 1/4 cup diced onions
- 1/4 cup shredded cheddar cheese.

1. Preheat oven to 350°F (175°C). Grease a muffin tin.
2. In a bowl, whisk the eggs.
3. Stir in the sausage, onions, and cheese.
4. Pour the mixture into the muffin tin.
5. Bake for 20-25 minutes.

Tips for Variation:

- Substitute the sausage with diced bell peppers, mushrooms, or spinach for a meat-free alternative.
- Experiment with different types of cheese such as mozzarella, feta, or pepper jack to enhance flavor.
- Add a pinch of smoked paprika, garlic powder, or Italian seasoning for extra flavor.

Nutritional Information: *Calories: 160, Fats: 12.7g, Protein: 10.3g, Carbs: 0.5g, Fiber: 0.1g, Sugar: 0g*

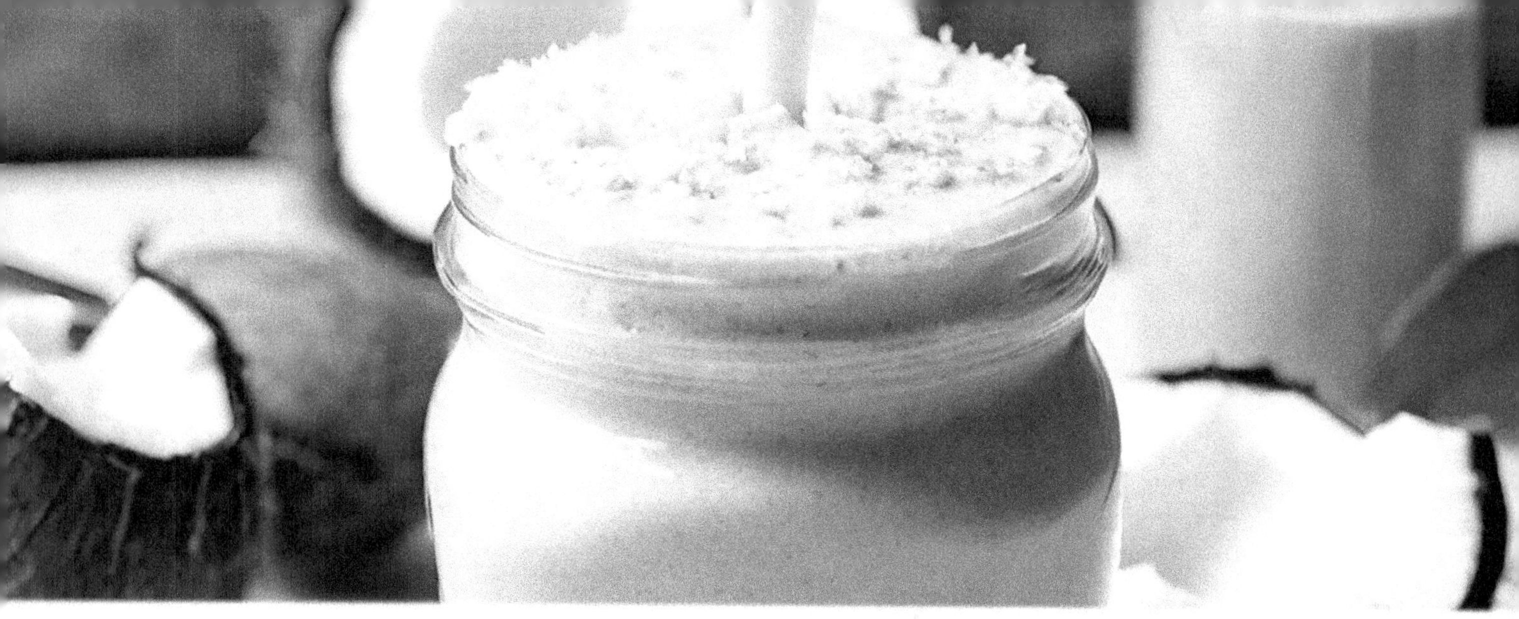

Vegan Keto Coconut Protein Shake

SERVINGS: 1   PREP TIME: 5 MINUTES   COOK TIME: 0 MINUTES

INGREDIENTS

- 1 cup Unsweetened Coconut Milk
- 1 ounce Protein Technologies International ProPlus Soy Protein Isolate
- 1/2 teaspoon Vanilla Extract

INSTRUCTIONS

1. Whey protein powder may be substituted (please add 1g NC additional to the total NC value) for non-vegans or vegetarians.
2. Combine all ingredients in a blender with 2-4 ice cubes (depending upon the thickness desired).
3. Consider adding coconut extract in addition to or instead of the vanilla.
4. Blend thoroughly and enjoy.

Tips for Variation:

- Add fresh or frozen berries for natural sweetness and extra nutrients.
- Nut Butter Twist: Mix in almond butter or peanut butter for creaminess and added protein.
- Green Power: Blend in spinach or kale for a nutritional boost without altering the taste.

Nutritional Information: *Protein: 24.4g, Fat: 5.6g, Fiber: 1g, Calories: 158.7, Net Carbs: 1.3g*

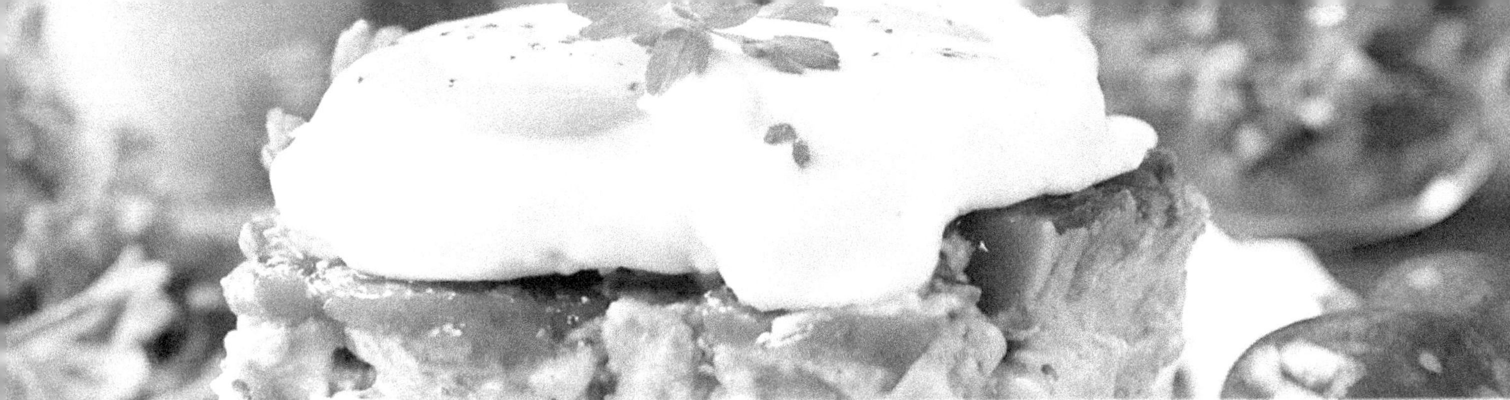

Turkey Breakfast Meatloaf Parfait

SERVINGS: 8   PREP TIME: 15 MINUTES   COOK TIME: 55 MINUTES

- 1 10 oz. package Frozen Chopped Spinach
- 4 stalks, medium (7-1/2" - 8" long) Celery
- 1 medium (approx. 2-3/4" long, 2-1/2" diameter) Sweet Red Peppers
- 24 ounces raw (yield after cooking) Turkey Breakfast Sausage
- 1 1/2 pounds Ground Turkey
- 6 large Eggs (Whole)
- 1 small Onion
- 1/2 tsp, ground Thyme (Dried)
- 1 medium (approx. 2-3/4" long, 2-1/2" diameter) Green Sweet Pepper
- 1/8 teaspoon Nutmeg (Ground)
- 1/8 tablespoon Red or Cayenne Pepper

1. Preheat oven to 350°F.
2. Thaw the spinach and coarsely chop.
3. Dice the celery, bell peppers, and white onion.
4. Combine the ground turkey sausage and turkey, spinach, celery, bell peppers, and onion until thoroughly mixed.
5. Add the eggs, thyme, cayenne, nutmeg, 1/2 teaspoon of garlic powder (if desired) and season with salt and freshly ground black pepper. Distribute evenly and place in two standard quick bread pans (4x9 inches).
6. Bake until cooked through and browned on top; about 55-65 minutes.
7. Serve immediately or freeze in individual portions for up to 2 months.

Tips for Variation:

- Try different herbs and spices like Italian seasoning or smoked paprika to customize the flavor.
- Sprinkle shredded cheese on top or layer it between the meat mixture for added richness.

Nutritional Information: *Calories: 340.4, Protein: 38.8g, Fat: 17.1g, Fiber: 2.4g, Net Carbs: 2.9g*

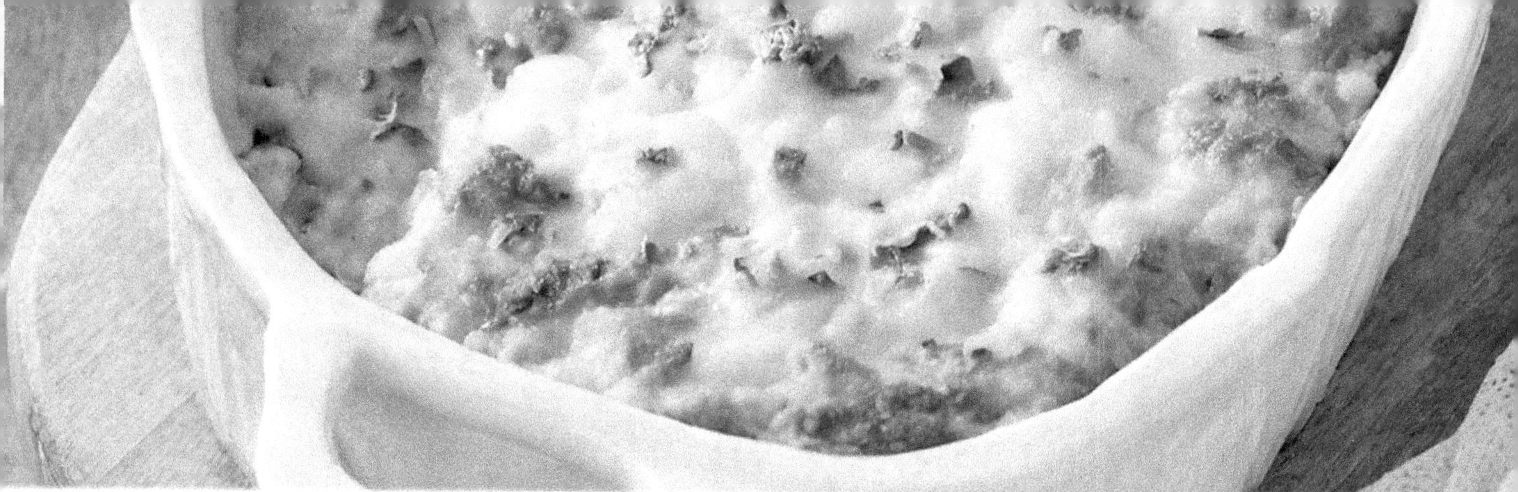

Egg Casserole

INGREDIENTS

- 6 eggs
- 1/2 cup cooked bacon
- 1/4 cup diced red and green bell peppers
- 1/4 cup shredded cheese.

INSTRUCTIONS

1. Preheat oven to 350°F (175°C).
2. In a bowl, whisk the eggs.
3. Stir in the bacon, bell peppers, and cheese.
4. Pour the mixture into a baking dish.
5. Bake for 20-25 minutes.

Tips for Variation:

- Add extra vegetables like spinach, mushrooms, or onions for added flavor and nutrition. Simply sauté them before adding to the egg mixture.
- Experiment with different proteins such as cooked sausage, ham, or turkey bacon instead of bacon for a different taste profile.
- Mix and match various types of cheese such as cheddar, mozzarella, or pepper jack to create a unique flavor combination. You can also sprinkle some grated Parmesan cheese on top for a crispy finish.

Nutritional Information: *Calories: 340.4, Protein: 38.8g, Fat: 17.1g, Fiber: 2.4g, Net Carbs: 2.9g*

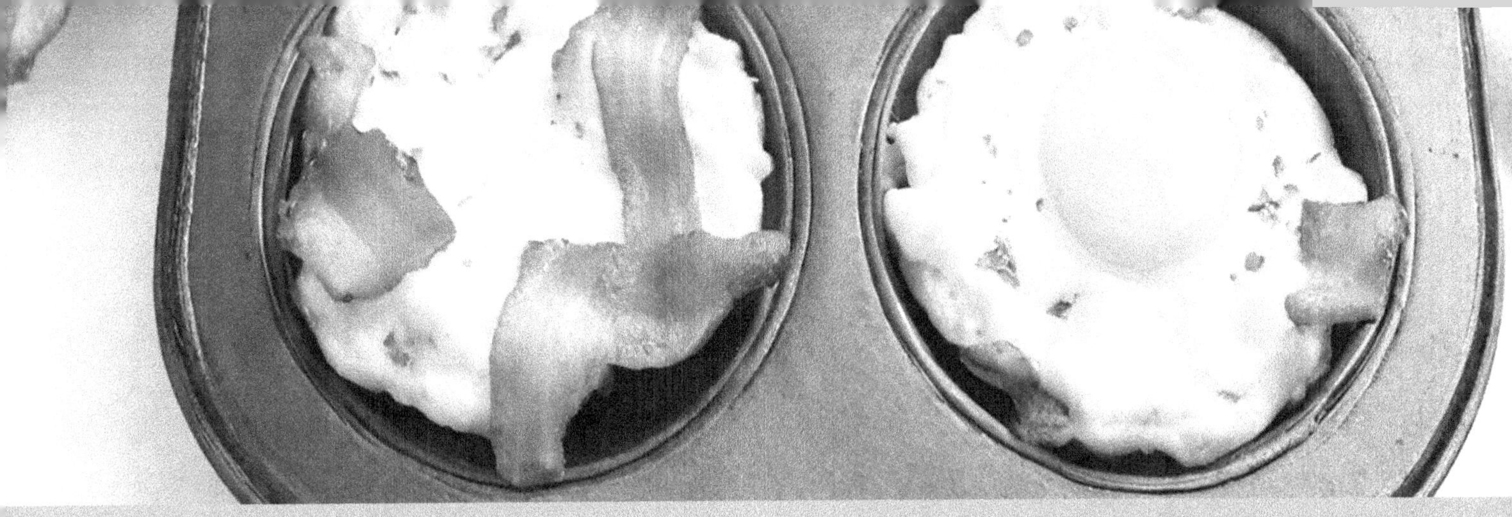

Bacon Egg Muffins

SERVINGS: 6   PREP TIME: 5 MINUTES   COOK TIME: 30 MINUTES

- 6 eggs
- 1/2 cup cooked bacon
- 1/4 cup diced green and red bell peppers
- 1/4 cup spinach
- 1/4 cup shredded cheese.

1. Preheat oven to 350°F (175°C).
2. Grease a muffin tin.
3. In a bowl, whisk the eggs.
4. Stir in the bacon, bell peppers, spinach, and cheese.
5. Pour the mixture into the muffin tin.
6. Bake for 20-25 minutes.

Tips for Variation:

- Experiment with different vegetables like diced tomatoes, onions, or mushrooms to add variety and nutrition to your muffins. You can also try adding jalapeños or diced zucchini for a flavorful twist.
- Enhance the flavor of your muffins by incorporating fresh herbs like chopped parsley, basil, or chives. These herbs not only add a burst of freshness but also elevate the overall taste of the dish.
- For a kick of flavor, add a pinch of spices such as garlic powder, paprika, or red pepper flakes to the egg mixture. Adjust the amount according to your taste preferences to create savory and satisfying muffins.

Nutritional Information: *Calories: 144, Fats: 11g, Protein: 10g, Net Carbs: 2g*

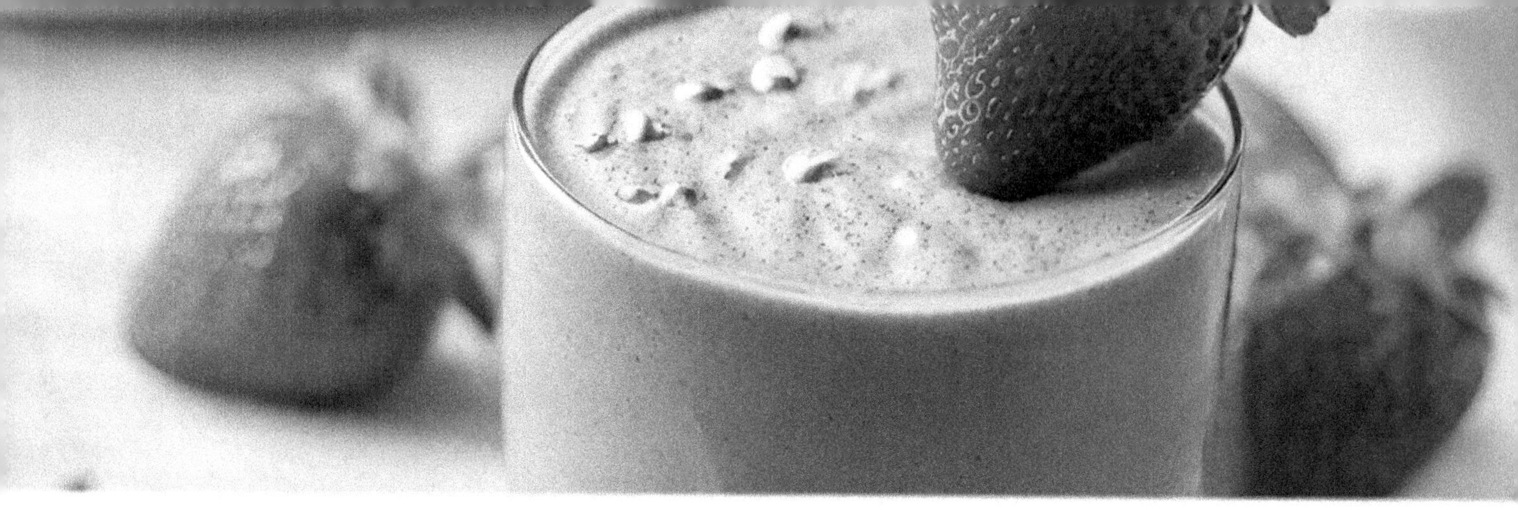

Chocolate & Strawberry Smoothie

SERVINGS: 1   PREP TIME: 5 MINUTES   COOK TIME: 0 MINUTES

INGREDIENTS

- 1 cup unsweetened almond milk (or any milk of your choice)
- 1 cup frozen strawberries
- 1 scoop chocolate protein powder
- 1 tablespoon unsweetened cocoa powder
- 1 tablespoon almond butter (or peanut butter)
- 1 teaspoon honey or low-carb sweetener (optional)
- Ice cubes (optional)

INSTRUCTIONS

1. Place all the ingredients in a blender.
2. Blend until smooth and creamy, adding more almond milk if needed to reach your desired consistency.
3. Taste and adjust sweetness by adding honey or sweetener if desired.
4. If you prefer a thicker smoothie, add some ice cubes and blend again until smooth.
5. Pour the smoothie into glasses and serve immediately.

Tips for Variation:

- Use fresh strawberries instead of frozen for a slightly different texture.
- Substitute the almond milk with coconut milk, soy milk, or dairy milk if preferred.
- Experiment with different flavors of protein powder such as vanilla or chocolate mint.

Nutritional Information: *Calories: 250 kcal, Total Fat: 10g, Saturated Fat: 1g, Cholesterol: 20mg, Sodium: 250mg, Total, Carbohydrates: 20g, Dietary Fiber: 6g, Sugars: 10g, Protein: 25g*

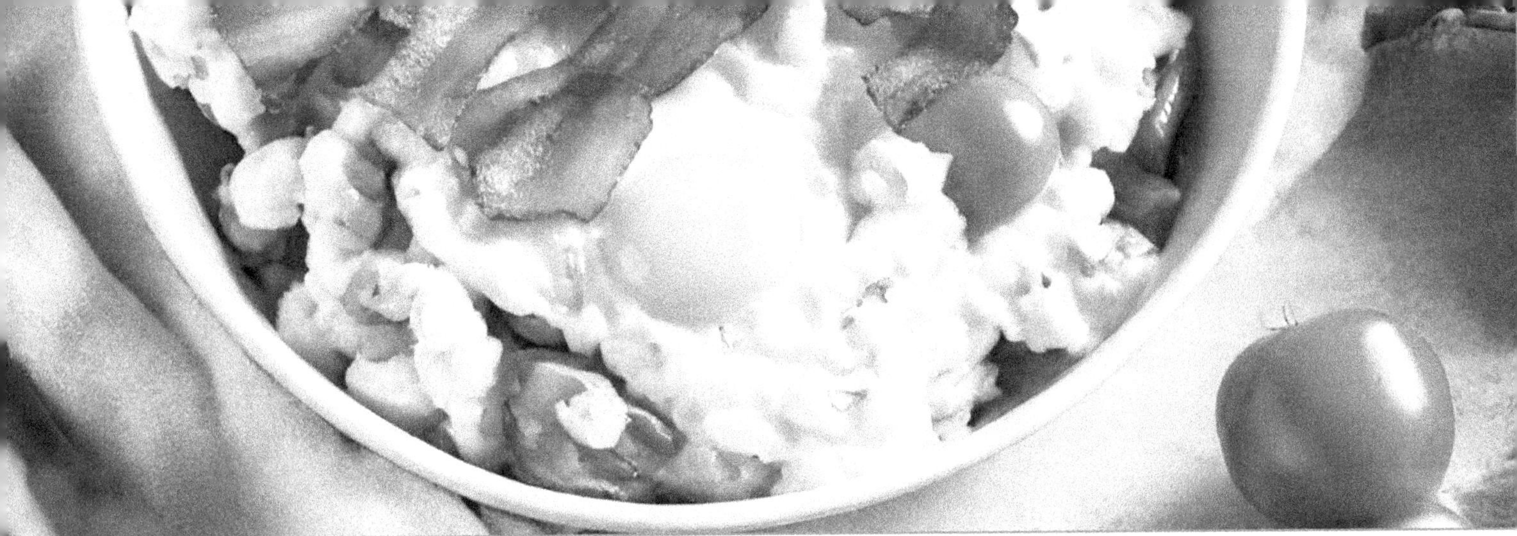

Scrambled Eggs with Bacon, Green Bell Peppers and Tomato

- 4 slices bacon, chopped
- 1/2 green bell pepper, diced
- 1 tomato, diced
- 6 large eggs
- Salt and pepper to taste
- 1 tablespoon butter or olive oil
- Optional garnish: chopped fresh parsley or chives

1. In a large skillet, cook the chopped bacon over medium heat until crispy. Remove the bacon from the skillet and set aside, leaving the bacon grease in the skillet.
2. In the same skillet with the bacon grease, add the diced green bell pepper and tomato. Cook for 3-4 minutes, or until the vegetables are softened.
3. While the vegetables are cooking, crack the eggs into a bowl and beat them lightly with a fork. Season with salt and pepper to taste.
4. Push the cooked vegetables to one side of the skillet and add the butter or olive oil to the empty side. Pour the beaten eggs into the skillet and let them cook undisturbed for a few seconds until the edges start to set.
5. Use a spatula to gently scramble the eggs, mixing them with the cooked vegetables.

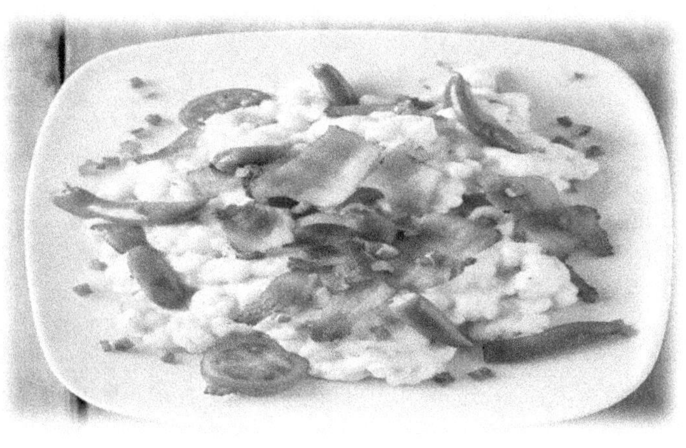

6. Continue cooking and stirring until the eggs are cooked to your desired consistency.

7. Once the eggs are cooked, stir in the cooked bacon pieces.

8. Remove the skillet from the heat and garnish with chopped fresh parsley or chives if desired.

9. Serve the scrambled eggs with bacon, green bell peppers, and tomato hot.

<u>Tips for Variation:</u>

- Add diced onions or mushrooms for extra flavor and texture.
- Use turkey bacon or Canadian bacon instead of regular bacon for a lower-fat option.
- Sprinkle shredded cheese on top of the scrambled eggs for added richness.
- Serve the scrambled eggs with whole grain toast or avocado slices for a complete meal.
- Experiment with different herbs and spices such as garlic powder, smoked paprika, or red pepper flakes to customize the flavor to your liking.

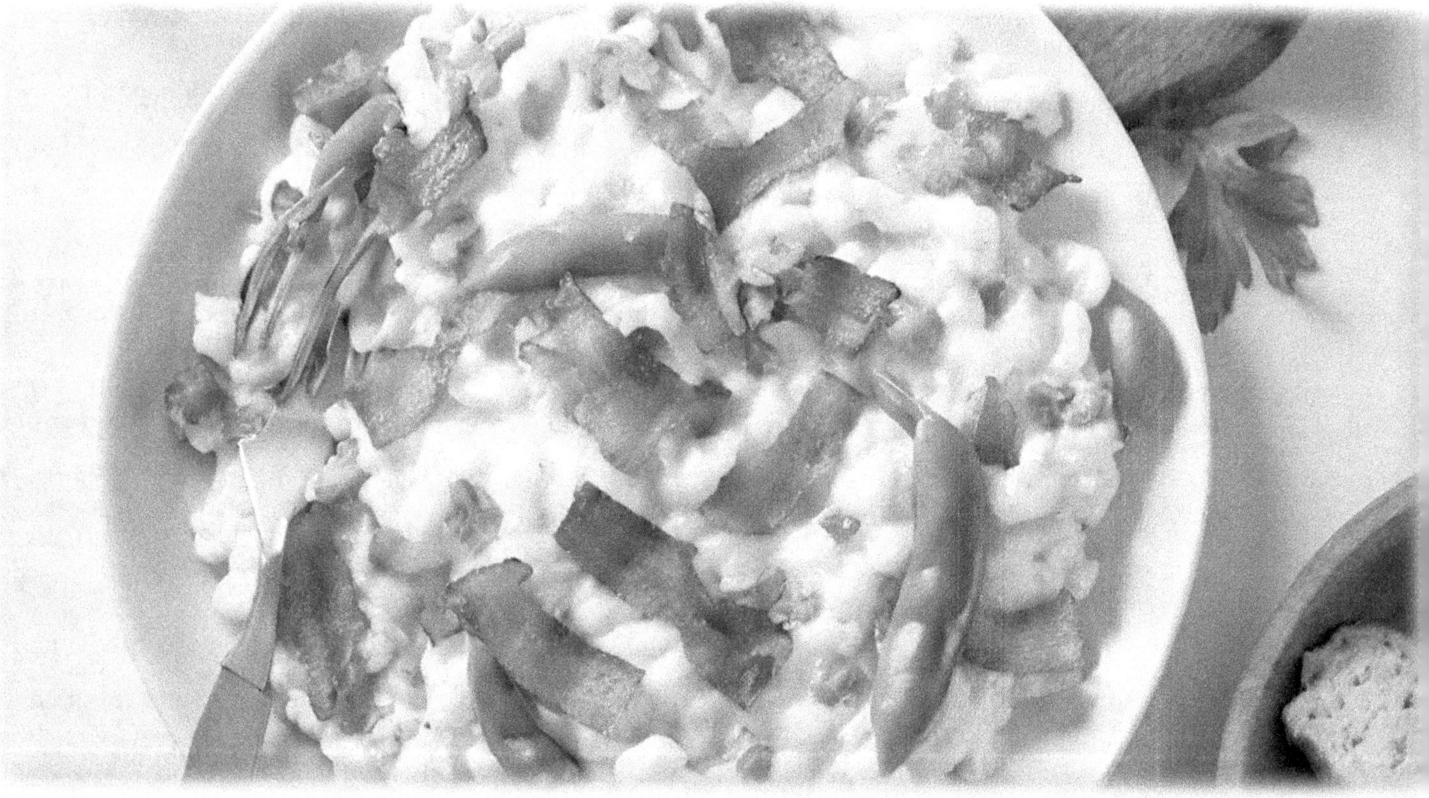

<u>Nutritional Information:</u> *Calories: 300 kcal, Total Fat: 22g, Saturated Fat: 8g, Cholesterol: 390mg, Sodium: 600mg, Total, Carbohydrates: 5g, Dietary Fiber: 1g, Sugars: 3g, Protein: 20g*

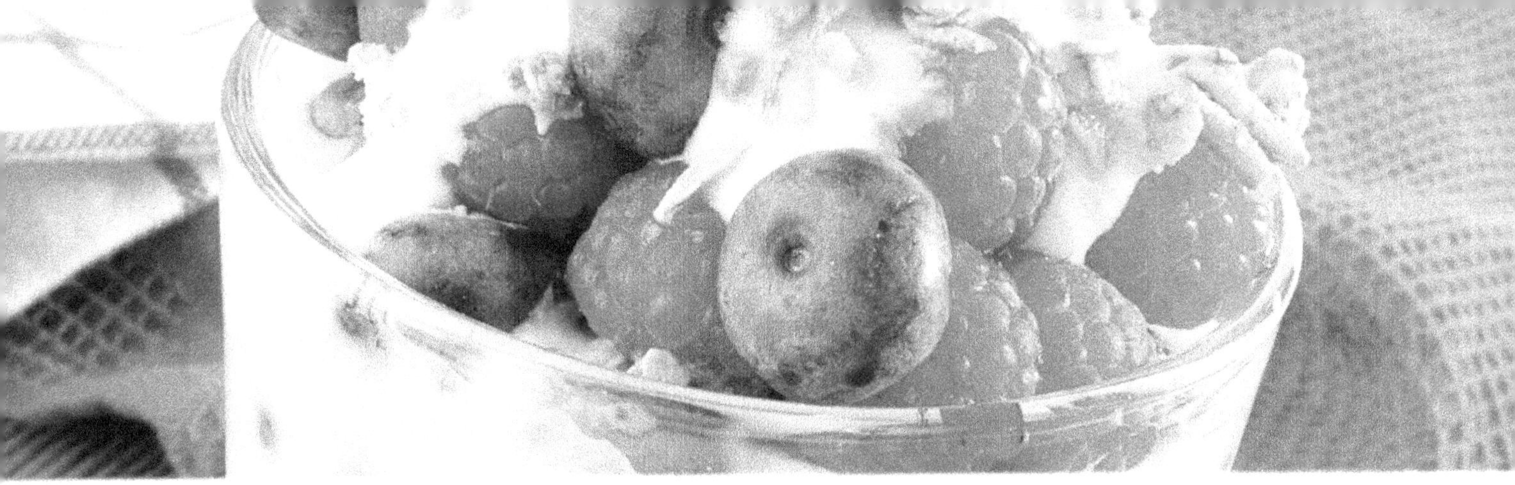

Berry Parfait

- 2 cups Raspberries
- 1 1/2 cup, wholes Strawberries
- 2 1/2 tablespoons Sucralose Based Sweetener (Sugar Substitute)
- 1 cup Heavy Cream
- 1 tablespoon Vanilla Extract
- 6 ounces Greek Yogurt - Plain (Container)
- 1 bar Atkins Strawberry Shortcake Bar

1. In a blender, purée 1 1/2 cups of the strawberries and 1 1/2 cups of the raspberries with 1 1/2 tablespoons sugar substitute.
2. In a large mixing bowl, with an electric mixer on medium speed, combine heavy cream, the remaining 1 tablespoon sugar substitute and the vanilla, beating to soft peaks.
3. Add yogurt (1 1/2 single serving containers) and beat to stiff peaks.
4. In four parfait glasses, alternate layers of the berry mixture, cream filling and crumbled Atkins bar, making at least two layers of each.
5. Top each with some of the remaining 1/2 cup raspberries and serve.

Tips for Variation:

Instead of using only raspberries and strawberries, mix in other berries like blueberries, blackberries, or sliced cherries for a diverse flavor profile and added antioxidants.

Nutritional Information: *Calories: 310 kcal, Total Fat: 25g, Saturated Fat: 15g, Cholesterol: 80mg, Sodium: 50mg, Total Carbohydrates: 20g, Dietary Fiber: 5g, Sugars: 10g, Protein: 4g*

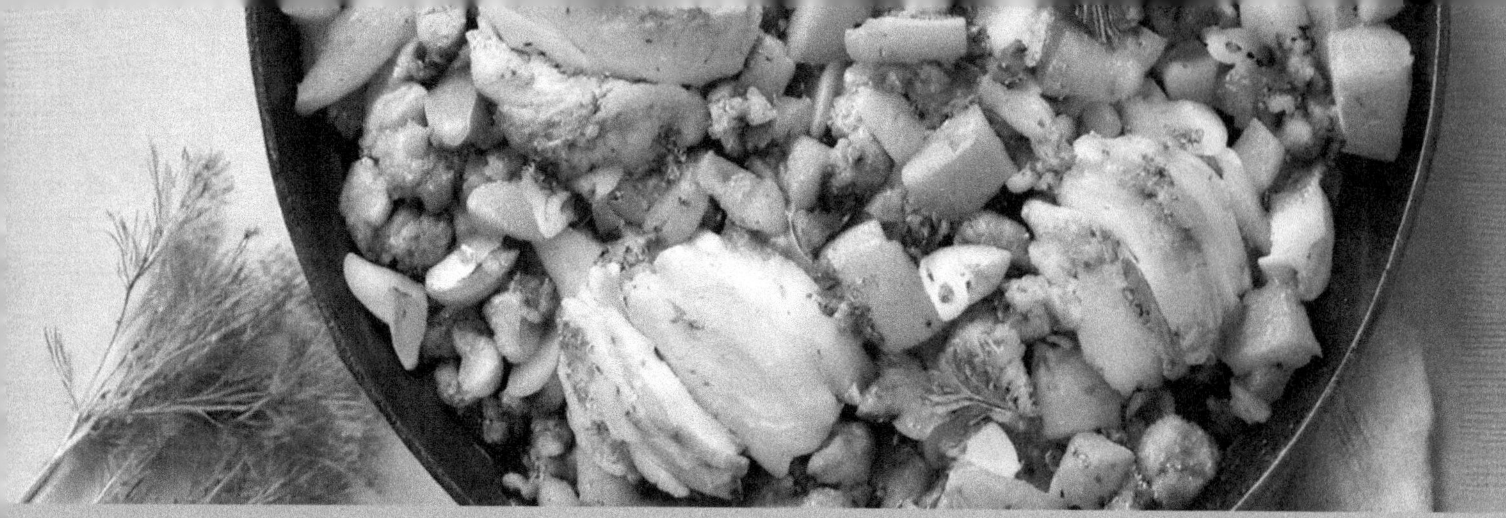

Fennel, Carrot and Turkey Hash

SERVINGS: 1   PREP TIME: 10 MINUTES   COOK TIME: 20 MINUTES

INGREDIENTS

- 2 tablespoons Canola Vegetable Oil
- 6 ounces Fennel Bulk
- 1/2 cup chopped Carrots
- 3 teaspoons Orange Zest
- 1/4 cup Freshly Squeezed Orange Juice
- 1/4 teaspoon Fennel Seed
- 1 tablespoon Tamari Soybean Sauce
- 1/2 cup chopped Scallions or Spring Onions1
- 12 ounces Turkey Breast Meat (Fryer-Roasters, Cooked, Roasted)

INSTRUCTIONS

1. Dice the fennel and carrot.
2. In a large skillet over medium heat, heat oil; add the fennel and carrot and sauté for about 3 minutes.
3. Zest and juice the orange.
4. Add orange zest and juice.
5. Simmer until liquid is almost absorbed, about 4 minutes.
6. Stir in fennel seeds, tamari, scallions and diced turkey.
7. Cook for another 6 minutes until the turkey is heated through.

Tips for Variation:

Enhance the flavor profile by adding fresh herbs such as thyme, rosemary, or sage to the hash. Simply chop the herbs finely and stir them in during the final minutes of cooking for a fragrant and savory twist.

Nutritional Information: *Calories: 350 kcal, Total Fat: 16g, Saturated Fat: 2g, Cholesterol: 70mg, Sodium: 350mg, Total Carbohydrates: 20g, Dietary Fiber: 7g, Sugars: 10g, Protein: 30g*

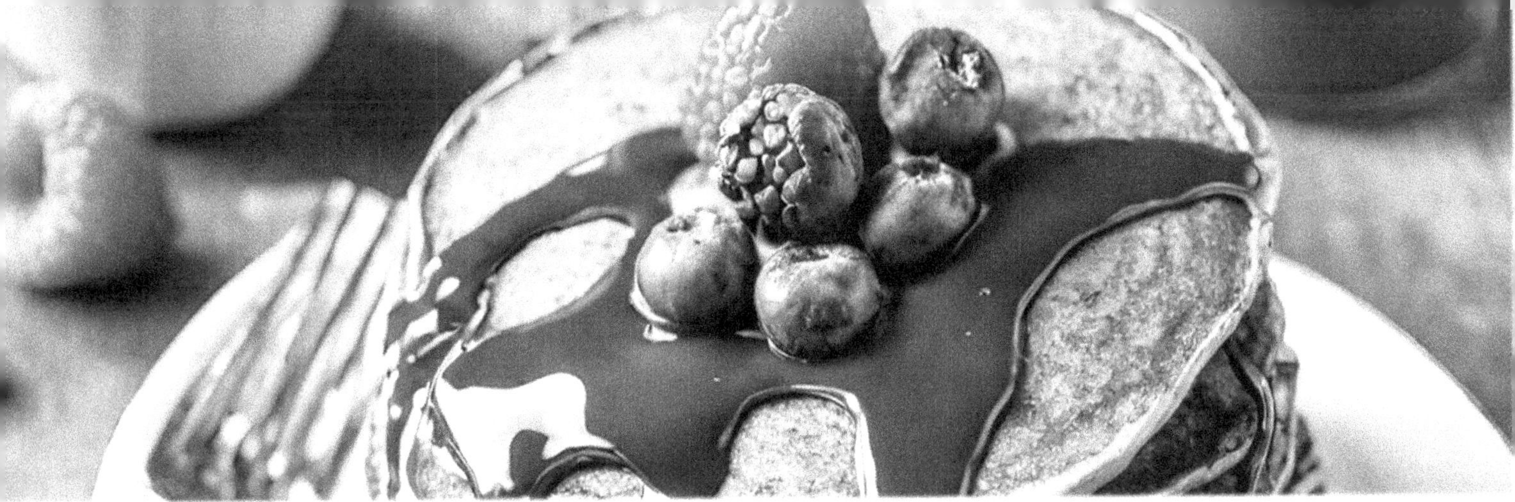

Chocolate Protein Pancakes

- 1/2 cup coconut flour
- 1/4 cup low-carb vanilla protein powder
- 1/4 cup unsweetened cocoa powder
- 2 eggs, 1/2 cup unsweetened almond milk.

1. In a bowl, mix the coconut flour, protein powder, and cocoa powder.
2. Stir in the eggs and almond milk until smooth. Heat a non-stick pan over medium heat.
3. Pour 1/4 cup of the batter onto the pan.
4. Cook until bubbles form on the surface, then flip and cook until browned on the other side.

Tips for Variation:

- Add a dollop of almond butter, peanut butter, or cashew butter to the pancake batter before cooking. Swirl it gently with a toothpick for a deliciously creamy and nutty flavor.
- Mix in chopped fresh berries like strawberries, raspberries, or blueberries to the batter for bursts of natural sweetness and added fiber. Fold the berries gently into the batter before cooking for even distribution.

Nutritional Information: *Calories: 200 kcal, Total Fat: 8g, Saturated Fat: 3g, Cholesterol: 190mg, Sodium: 200mg, Total Carbohydrates: 15g, Dietary Fiber: 8g, Sugars: 2g, Protein: 18g*

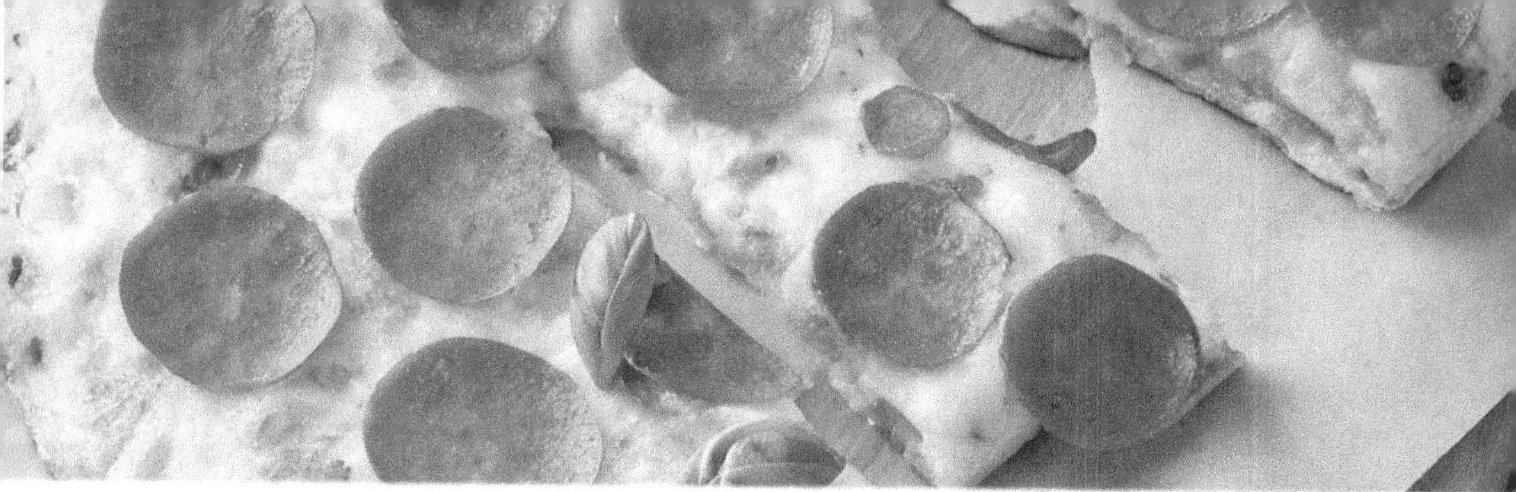

Pepperoni Pizza Frittata

SERVINGS: 6   PREP TIME: 5 MINUTES   COOK TIME: 15 MINUTES

INGREDIENTS

- 6 eggs
- 1/2 cup pepperoni slices
- 1/4 cup diced green peppers
- 1/4 cup basil leaves
- 1/4 cup tomato sauce.

INSTRUCTIONS

1. Preheat oven to 350°F (175°C).
2. In a bowl, whisk the eggs.
3. Stir in the pepperoni, green peppers, basil leaves, and tomato sauce.
4. Pour the mixture into a baking dish.
5. Bake for 20-25 minutes.

Tips for Variation:

- Amp up the pizza flavor by adding a blend of shredded mozzarella, Parmesan, or cheddar cheese to the egg mixture. Sprinkle it over the top before baking for a gooey and melty cheese layer.
- For a vegetarian option, omit the pepperoni and add a variety of sautéed vegetables like mushrooms, onions, or spinach. Customize the frittata with your favorite pizza veggies.

Nutritional Information: Calories: 120 kcal, Total Fat: 8g, Saturated Fat: 3g, Cholesterol: 220mg, Sodium: 250mg, Total Carbohydrates: 3g, Dietary Fiber: 1g, Sugars: 1g, Protein: 10g

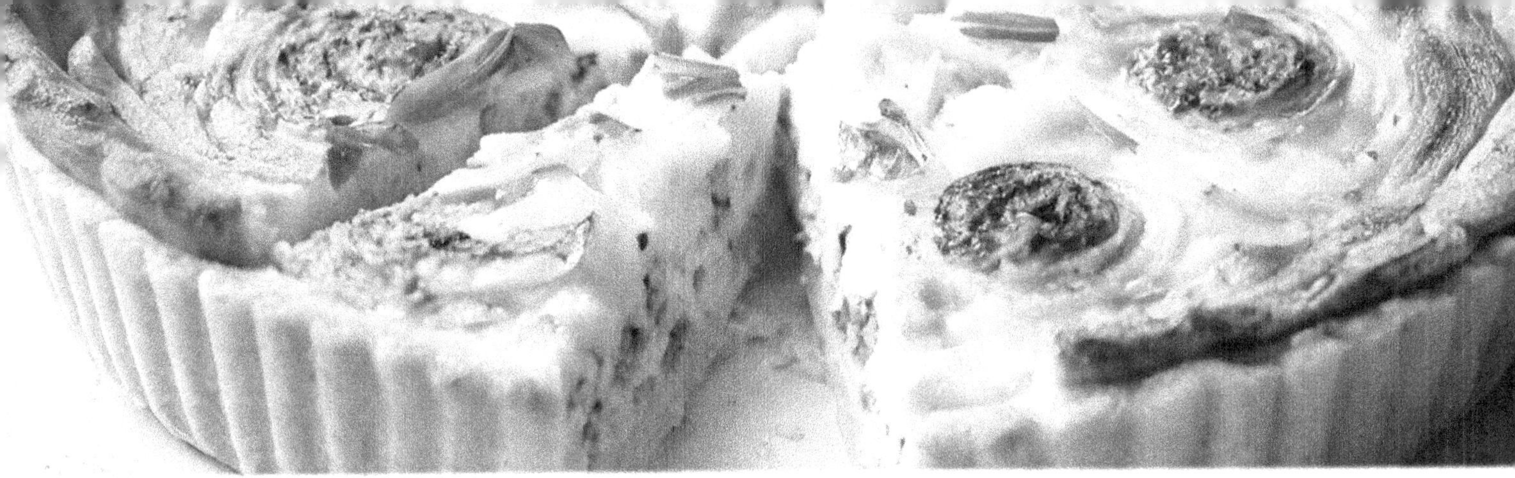

Leek Quiche

- 8 servings Atkins Pie Crust
- 1 tablespoon Unsalted Butter Stick
- 1 1/2 pounds Leeks
- 1/2 cup Heavy Cream
- 3 large Eggs (Whole)
- 1/2 teaspoon Salt
- 1/4 teaspoon Black Pepper
- 1 cup shredded Gruyere Cheese

<u>Tips for Variation:</u>

Add a burst of freshness and flavor by incorporating chopped fresh herbs such as thyme, parsley, or chives into the egg mixture before baking. These herbs will complement the leeks beautifully and elevate the overall taste of the quiche.

1. Prebake the shell and pour filling (directions follow) into hot shell. Keep oven on at 350°F.
2. In a medium skillet over medium heat, melt butter. Add diced leeks and sauté, stirring occasionally, 5 to 6 minutes, until softened.
3. Remove from heat and stir in cream. Let stand 5 minutes.
4. Meanwhile, in a medium bowl, whisk eggs with salt and pepper.
5. Stir egg mixture into the leeks and cream.
6. Sprinkle ¾ cup of cheese on bottom of pie shell.
7. Pour egg mixture into prebaked pie shell; sprinkle remaining cheese on top.
8. Bake 45 minutes, or until just set in middle and browned on top.
9. If necessary, turn on broiler; broil 6 from element 2 minutes, just until top browns.

<u>**Nutritional Information:**</u> *Calories: 300 kcal, Total Fat: 20g, Saturated Fat: 10g, Cholesterol: 140mg, Sodium: 400mg, Total Carbohydrates: 20g, Dietary Fiber: 2g, Sugars: 2g, Protein: 12g*

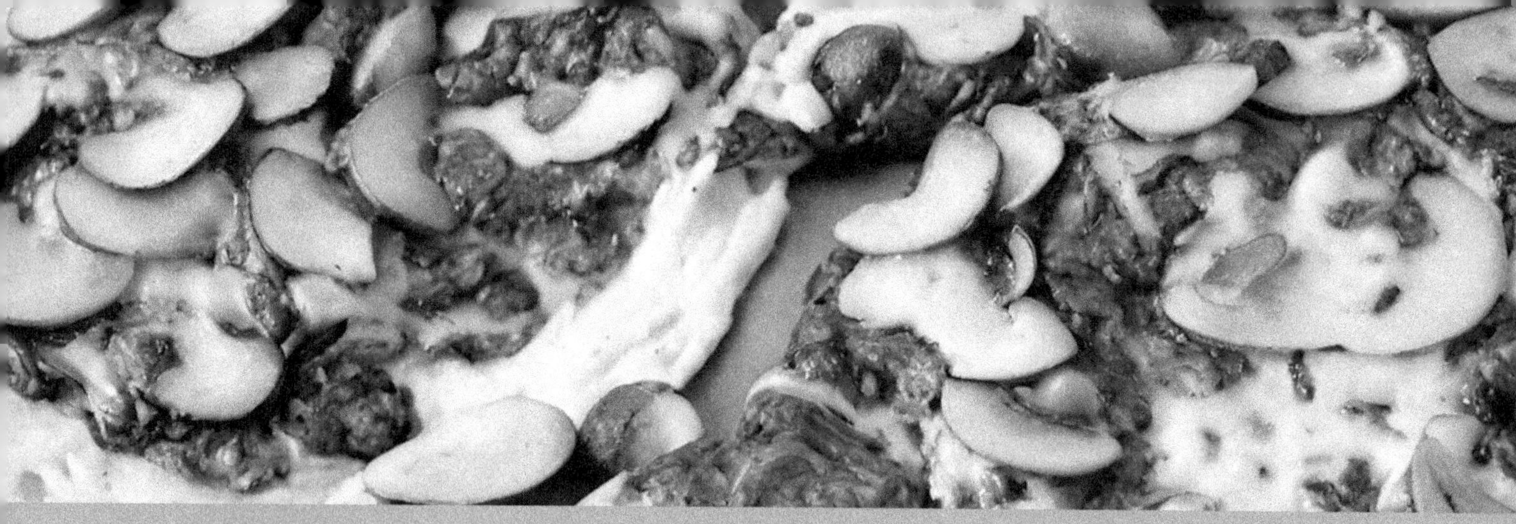

Spinach and Mushroom Omelette

SERVINGS: 2   PREP TIME: 5 MINUTES   COOK TIME: 10 MINUTES

INGREDIENTS

- 4 large eggs
- 1 cup fresh spinach leaves, chopped
- 1/2 cup sliced mushrooms
- 1/4 cup shredded cheese (such as cheddar, mozzarella, or feta)
- Salt and pepper to taste
- 1 tablespoon olive oil or butter

INSTRUCTIONS

1. In a mixing bowl, beat the eggs until well combined. Season with salt and pepper to taste.

2. Heat the olive oil or butter in a non-stick skillet over medium heat.

3. Add the chopped spinach and sliced mushrooms to the skillet. Cook for 2-3 minutes, stirring occasionally, until the vegetables are softened.

4. Pour the beaten eggs over the cooked vegetables in the skillet. Allow the eggs to set slightly around the edges.

5. Using a spatula, gently lift the edges of the omelette and tilt the skillet to let the uncooked eggs flow to the edges.

6. Once the omelette is mostly set but still slightly runny on top, sprinkle the shredded cheese evenly over one half of the omelette.

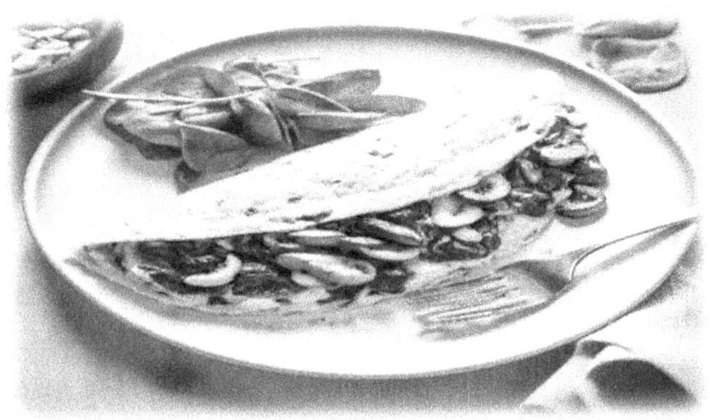

7. Carefully fold the other half of the omelette over the cheese to form a half-moon shape. Press down gently with the spatula to seal.

8. Cook for another 1-2 minutes until the cheese is melted and the omelette is cooked through.

9. Slide the omelette onto a plate and serve hot.

Tips for Variation:

- Customize your omelette by adding other vegetables such as bell peppers, onions, tomatoes, or zucchini.

- Incorporate cooked diced chicken, turkey, ham, or bacon for added protein and flavor.

- Spice it Up: Add a pinch of red pepper flakes or a dash of hot sauce for a spicy kick.

- Enhance the flavor with chopped fresh herbs like parsley, basil, or chives.

- Omit the cheese for a dairy-free version or substitute with dairy-free cheese alternatives.

- Mediterranean Twist: Replace the mushrooms with sun-dried tomatoes, Kalamata olives, and crumbled feta cheese for a Mediterranean-inspired omelette.

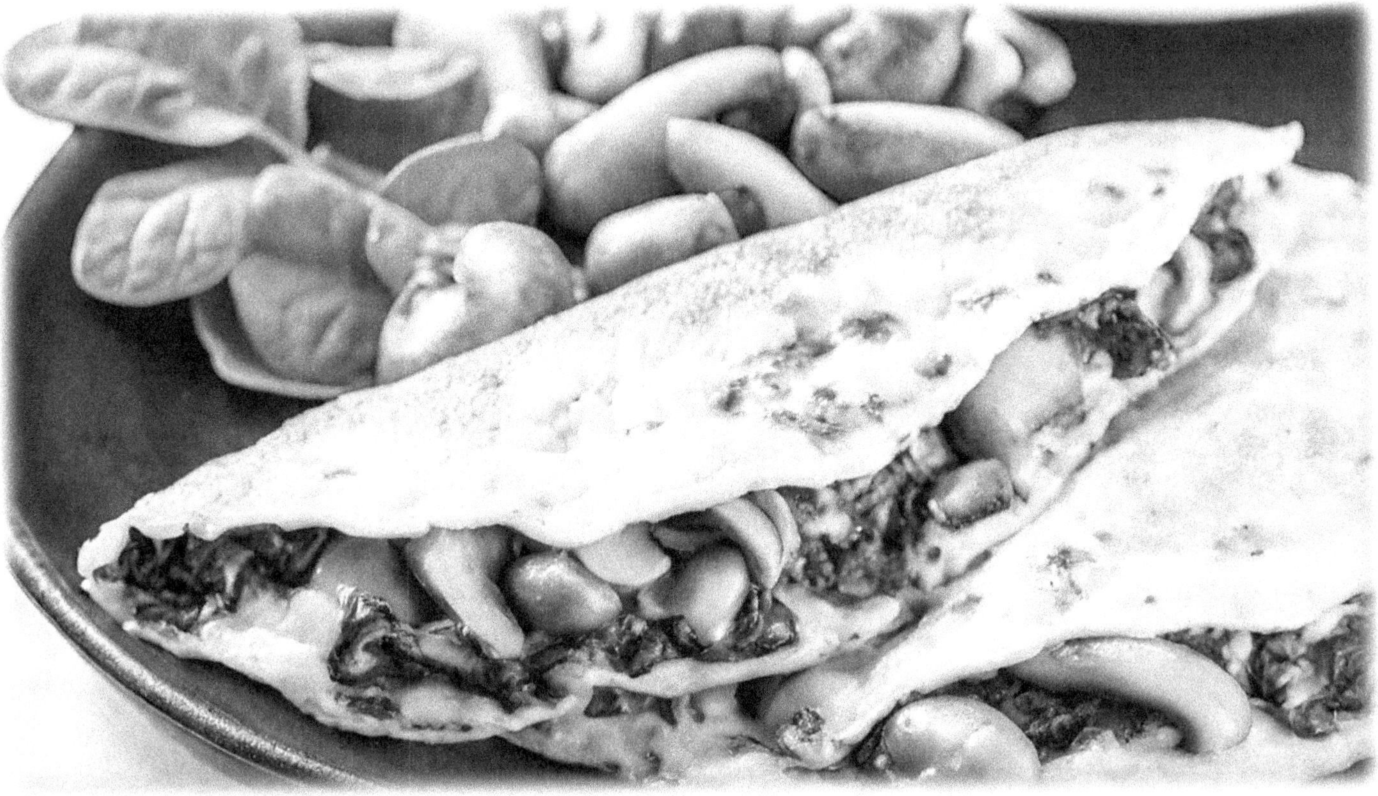

Nutritional Information: *Calories: 250 kcal, Total Fat: 19g, Saturated Fat: 7g, Cholesterol: 380mg, Sodium: 350mg, Total Carbohydrates: 4g, Dietary Fiber: 1g, Sugars: 1g, Protein: 17g*

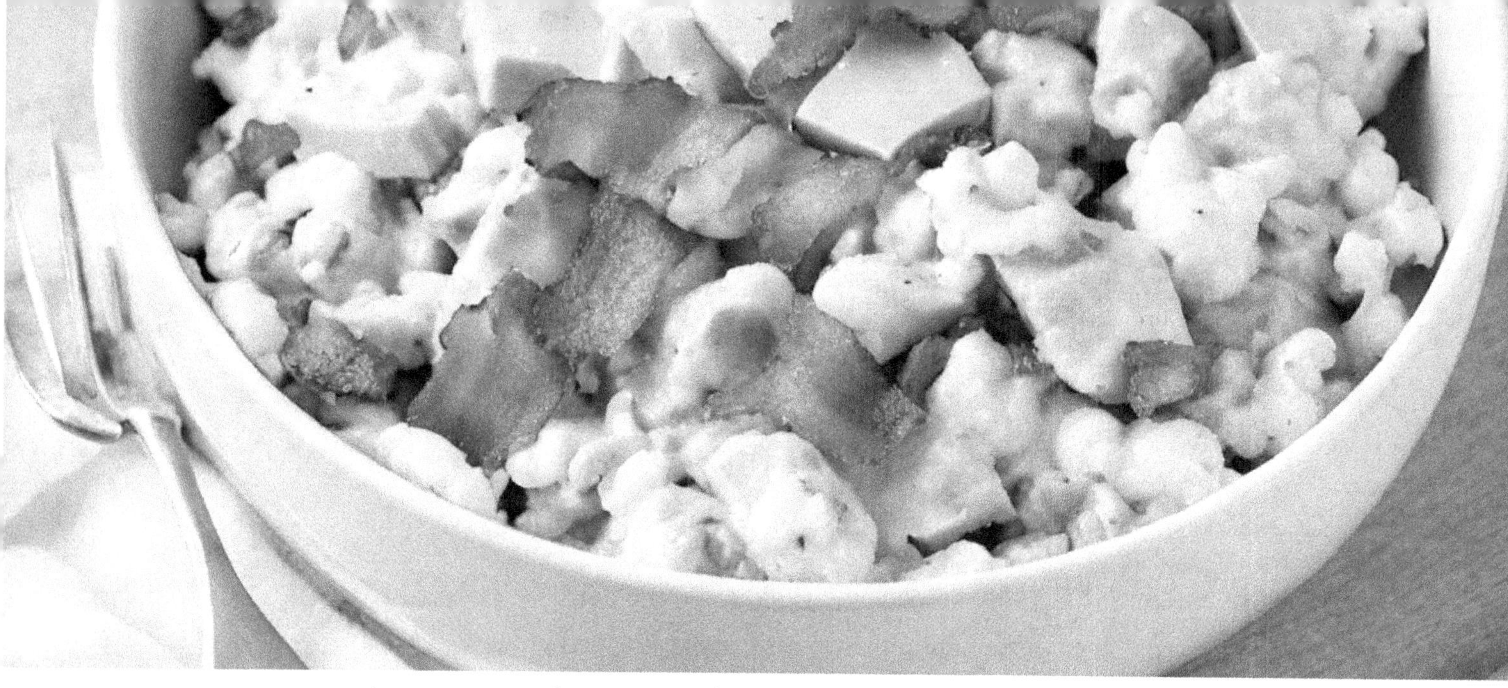

Avocado and Bacon Scramble

SERVINGS: 2   PREP TIME: 5 MINUTES   COOK TIME: 10 MINUTES

INGREDIENTS

- Ingredients:
- 4 slices bacon, chopped
- 4 large eggs
- 1 ripe avocado, diced
- Salt and pepper to taste
- Optional toppings: chopped fresh parsley, shredded cheese, hot sauce

INSTRUCTIONS

1. In a non-stick skillet, cook the chopped bacon over medium heat until crispy. Remove the bacon from the skillet and set aside, leaving the bacon grease in the skillet.

2. In a mixing bowl, beat the eggs until well combined. Season with salt and pepper to taste.

3. Pour the beaten eggs into the skillet with the bacon grease. Cook over medium heat, stirring occasionally, until the eggs are scrambled to your desired consistency.

4. Once the eggs are cooked, add the diced avocado to the skillet. Stir gently to combine with the scrambled eggs and warm the avocado slightly.

5. Sprinkle the cooked bacon pieces over the avocado and egg mixture.

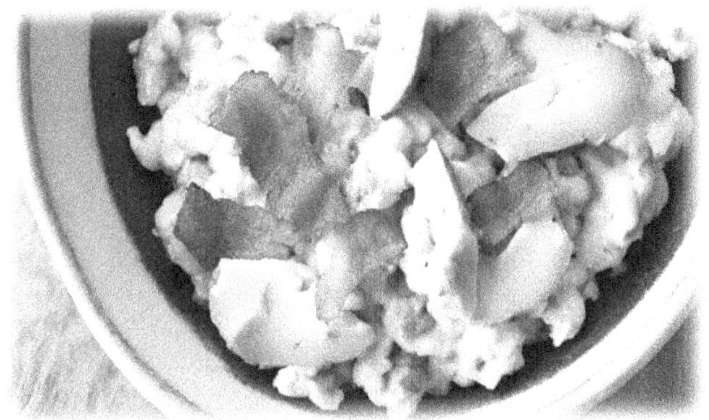

6. Serve the avocado and bacon scramble hot, garnished with optional toppings like chopped fresh parsley, shredded cheese, or hot sauce.

Tips for Variation:

- Omit the bacon and add diced sautéed vegetables like bell peppers, onions, or mushrooms for a vegetarian version of the scramble.
- Sprinkle shredded cheese like cheddar, Monterey Jack, or feta over the scrambled eggs and let it melt for added creaminess and flavor.
- Mix in chopped fresh herbs such as cilantro, basil, or dill to the scrambled eggs for a burst of freshness and aroma.
- Add a pinch of paprika, cayenne pepper, or chili flakes for a spicy kick. Alternatively, serve the scramble with your favorite hot sauce for extra heat

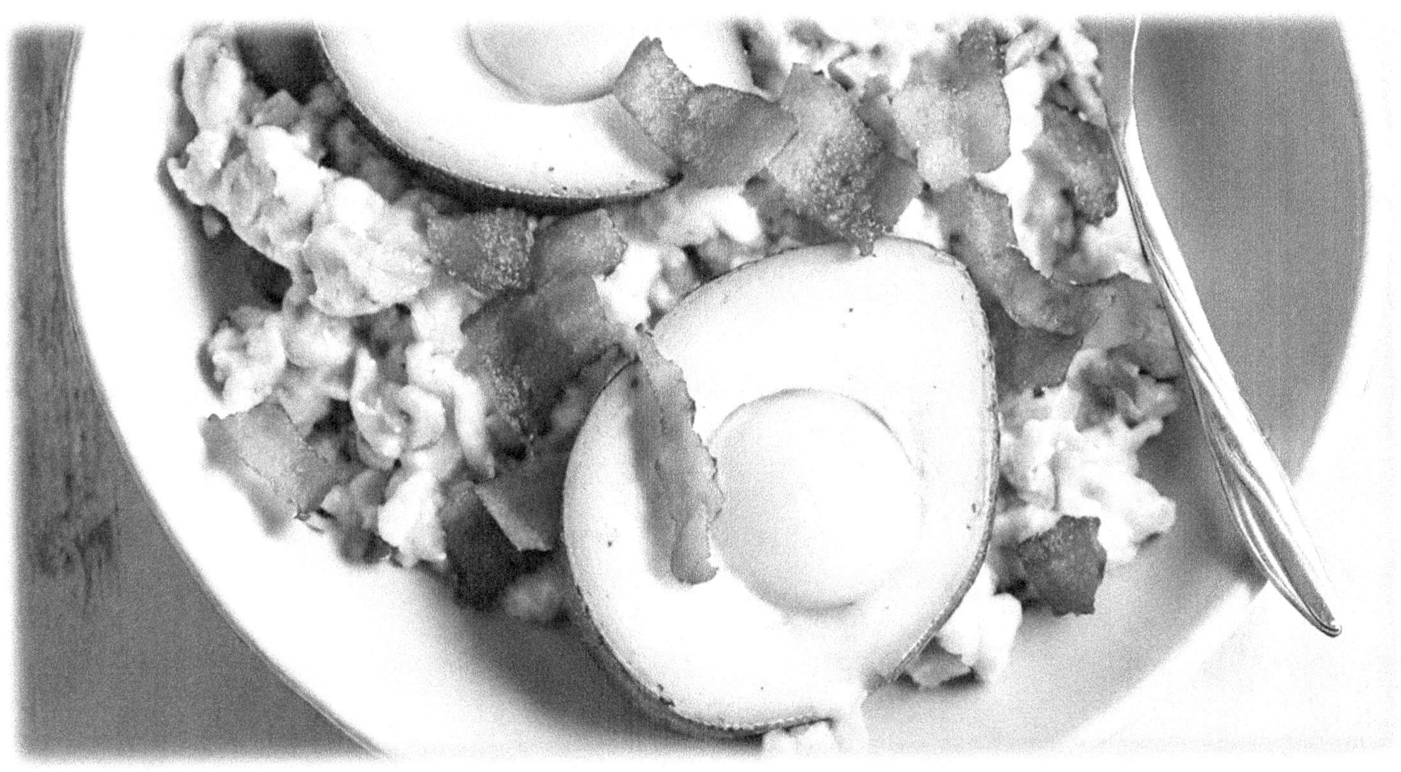

Nutritional Information: *Calories: 320 kcal, Total Fat: 25g, Saturated Fat: 7g, Cholesterol: 375mg, Sodium: 400mg, Total Carbohydrates: 5g, Dietary Fiber: 3g, Sugars: 0g, Protein: 20g*

Notes:

Your
Observation:

Progress
Report:

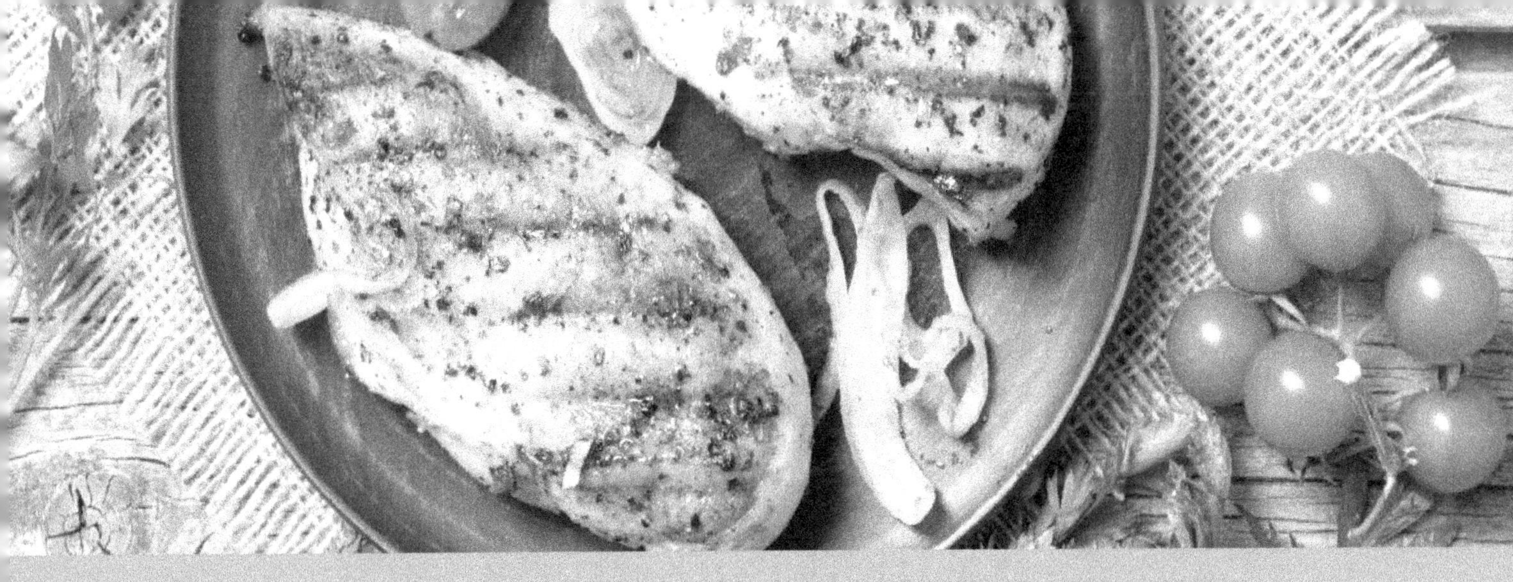

Phase 1: Induction Recipes

Three-Style Chicken Breast

SERVINGS: 1   PREP TIME: 10 MINUTES   COOK TIME: 20 TO 25 MINUTES

- 3 chicken breasts
- Salt and black pepper
- Garlic
- Lime and parsley

1. Season each chicken breast differently: one with salt and black pepper, one with garlic, and one with lime and parsley.
2. Grill each chicken breast separately.
3. Ensure the chicken is thoroughly cooked and no longer pink in the center.

<u>Tips for Variation:</u>

- Adjust seasonings to taste.
- Brine chicken breasts before grilling for a juicier result.
- Flatten chicken breasts to a uniform thickness for even cooking.
- Let the chicken rest after grilling to redistribute juices.

<u>Nutritional Information (per 3-ounce serving):</u> *Calories: 128, Fats: 2.7g, Protein: 26g, Carbs: 0g, Fiber: 0g, Sugar: 0g*

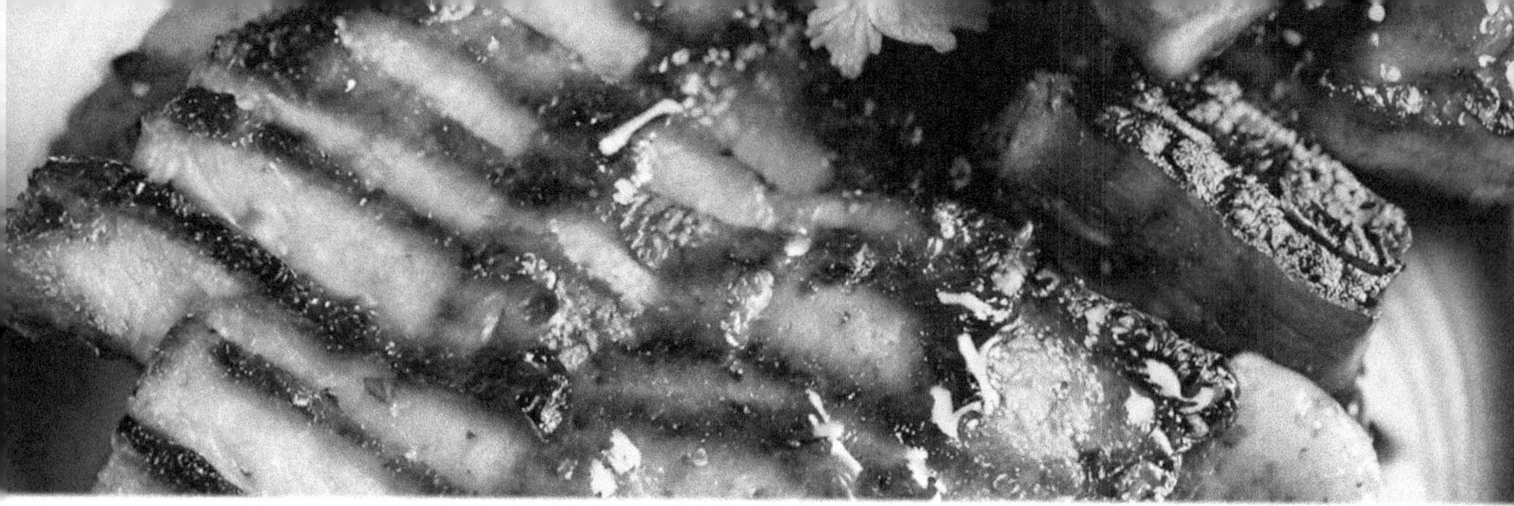

Grilled Pork Belly

SERVINGS: 4   PREP TIME: 1 HOUR   COOK TIME: 25 MINUTES

INGREDIENTS

- 3 lbs. pork belly
- 3/4 cup soy sauce
- Juice of 5 pieces lime
- 1 tablespoon garlic powder
- 1/4 tablespoon ground black pepper
- 1 teaspoon sriracha sauce or hot sauce

INSTRUCTIONS

1. Combine the soy sauce, lime juice, ground black pepper, garlic powder, and hot sauce in a large bowl.
2. Put the cleaned pork belly in a large resealable bag.
3. Pour the soy sauce mixture in the resealable bag.
4. Let the pork belly marinate for at least 1 hour.
5. Heat-up the grill.
6. Start to grill the marinated pork belly for 3 minutes per side.
7. Baste the pork belly with the remaining marinade.

Tips for Variation:

- Don't rush the marinade, but don't overdo it.
- You want to flip the pork belly slab over every 3 minutes, and baste it with marinade every single time.
- We're using skin-on pork belly for this recipe, but you can use skinless pork belly if you prefer it.

Nutritional Information: *Calories: 766, Fats: 72g, Protein: 14g, Carbs: 15g, Fiber: 0.2g, Sugar: 14g*

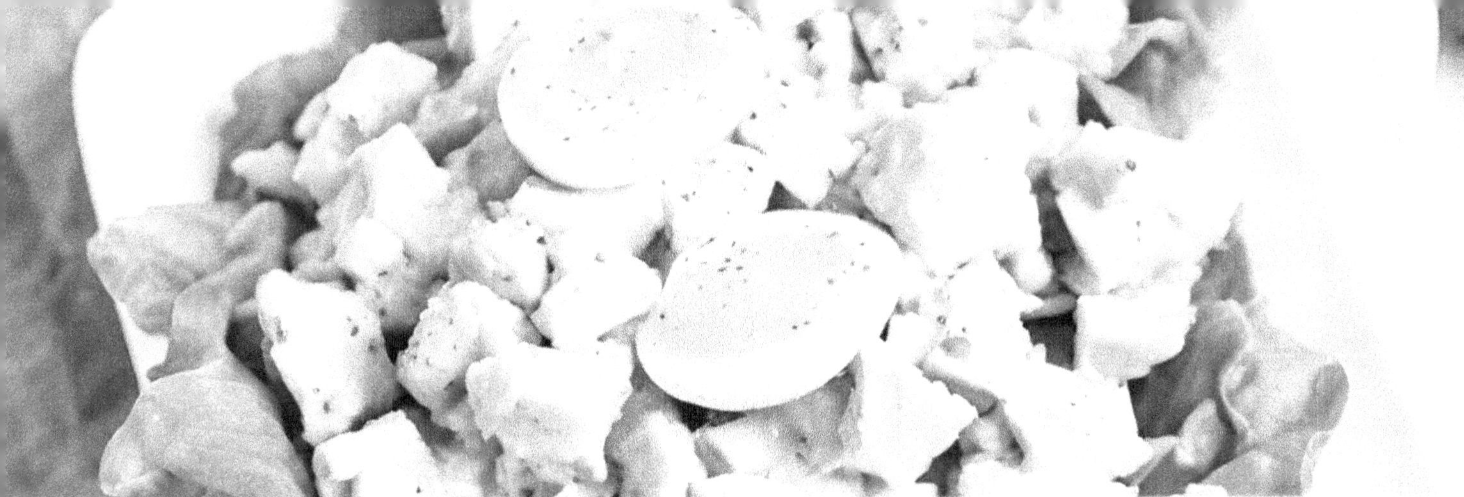

Avocado Egg Salad

- 1 Medium Avocado (pitted and peeled)
- 2 tablespoons Light Mayonnaise (or Greek yogurt)
- 1 ½ teaspoons Fresh Lemon Juice
- 4 Hard-Boiled Eggs (peeled and chopped)
- 1 Medium-Length Celery Stalk (finely chopped, about 3 tablespoons)
- 1 tablespoon Chives (finely chopped, parsley or dill)
- Salt And Fresh Ground Black Pepper

1. Mash the avocado with a tiny bit of mayonnaise in a bowl until it's creamy.
2. Stir in the chopped hard-boiled eggs, celery, lemon juice, and herbs.
3. Season with salt and pepper to taste.

<u>Tips for Variation:</u>

- If you want to keep this mayo-free, no problem, just leave it out or substitute with plain yogurt.
- When you stir everything together, try to keep things a little chunky.

<u>Nutritional Information:</u> *Calories: 269 kcal, Fats: 21g, Protein: 11g, Carbs: 3g, Fiber: 3g, Sugar: 2g*

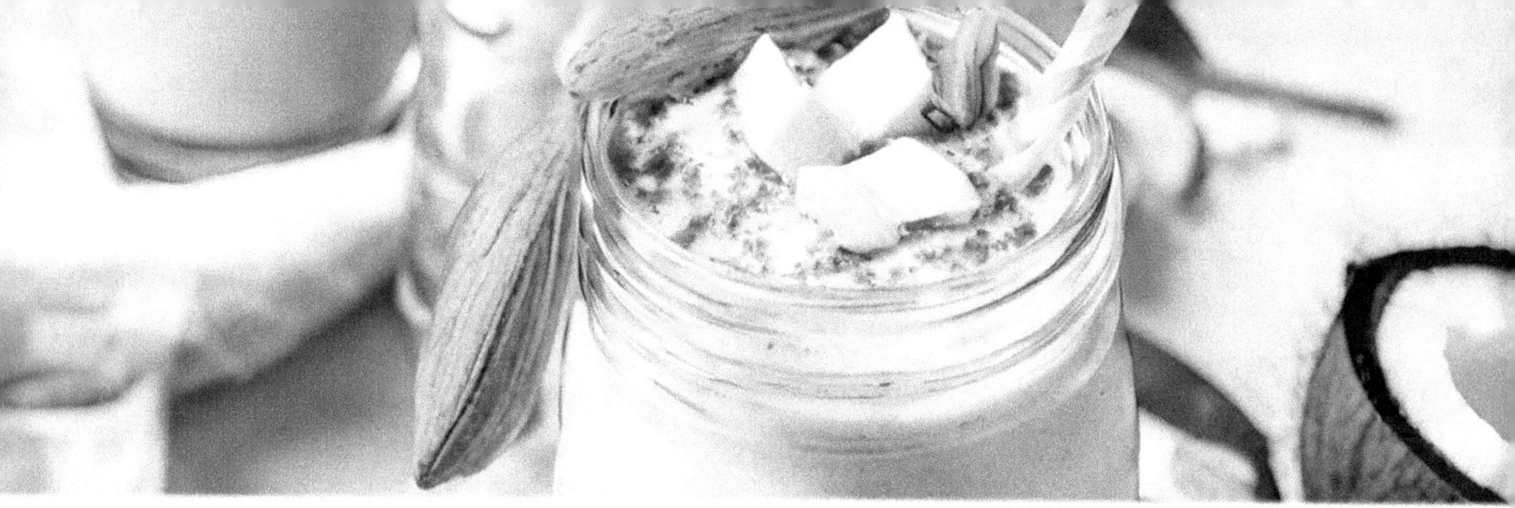

Vegan Keto Coconut Protein Shake

SERVINGS: 1   PREP TIME: 5 MINUTES   COOK TIME: 0 MINUTES

INGREDIENTS

- 1 cup of Unsweetened Coconut Milk
- 1 ounce of Protein Technologies International ProPlus Soy Protein Isolate
- 1/2 teaspoon of Vanilla Extract

INSTRUCTIONS

1. Combine all ingredients in a blender with 2-4 ice cubes (depending upon the thickness desired).
2. Consider adding coconut extract in addition to or instead of the vanilla.
3. Blend thoroughly and enjoy.

Tips for Variation:

- Whey protein powder may be substituted (please add 1g NC additional to the total NC value) for non-vegans or vegetarians.
- You could consider adding coconut extract in addition to or instead of the vanilla for a different flavor profile.

Nutritional Information: *Calories: 158.7cal, Protein: 24.4g, Fat: 5.6g, Fiber: 1g, Net Carbs: 1.3g, Sugar: N/A*

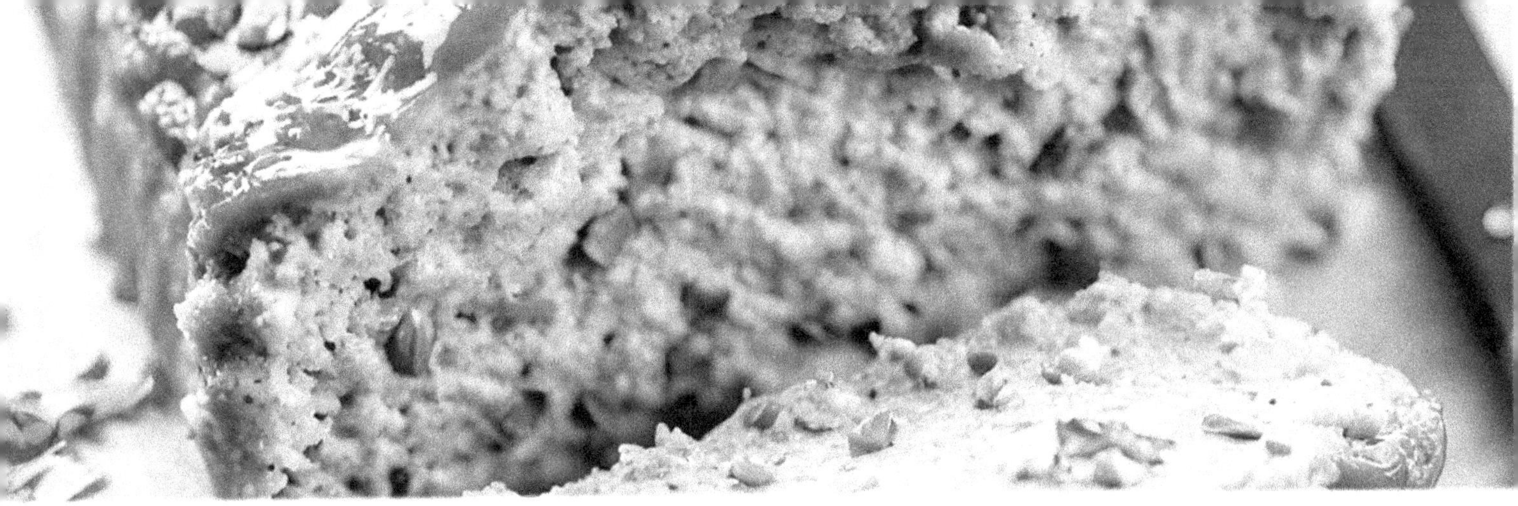

Keto Turkey Meatloaf

- 1 10 oz. package Frozen Chopped Spinach
- 4 stalk, medium (7-1/2" - 8" long) Celery
- 1 medium (approx. 2-3/4" long, 2-1/2" diameter) Sweet Red Peppers
- 24-ounce raw (yield after cooking) Turkey Breakfast Sausage
- 1 1/2 pounds Ground Turkey
- 6 large Eggs (Whole)
- 1 small Onion
- 1/2 tsp, ground Thyme (Dried)
- 1 medium (approx. 2-3/4" long, 2-1/2" diameter) Green Sweet Pepper
- 1/8 teaspoon Nutmeg (Ground)
- 1/8 tablespoon Red or Cayenne Pepper

1. Preheat oven to 350°F.
2. Thaw the spinach and coarsely chop.
3. Dice the celery, bell peppers, and white onion.
4. Combine the ground turkey sausage and turkey, spinach, celery, bell peppers, and onion until thoroughly mixed.
5. Add the eggs, thyme, cayenne, nutmeg, 1/2 teaspoon of garlic powder (if desired), and season with salt and freshly ground black pepper.
6. Distribute evenly and place in two standard quick bread pans (4x9 inches).
7. Bake until cooked through and browned on top; about 55-65 minutes.
8. Serve immediately or freeze in individual portions for up to 2 months.

- One of the things I love the most about this recipe is that it's highly customizable. You can add or subtract any ingredients depending on your preferences. For example, you can add some chopped vegetables like carrots or zucchini to the mixture for added nutrition.

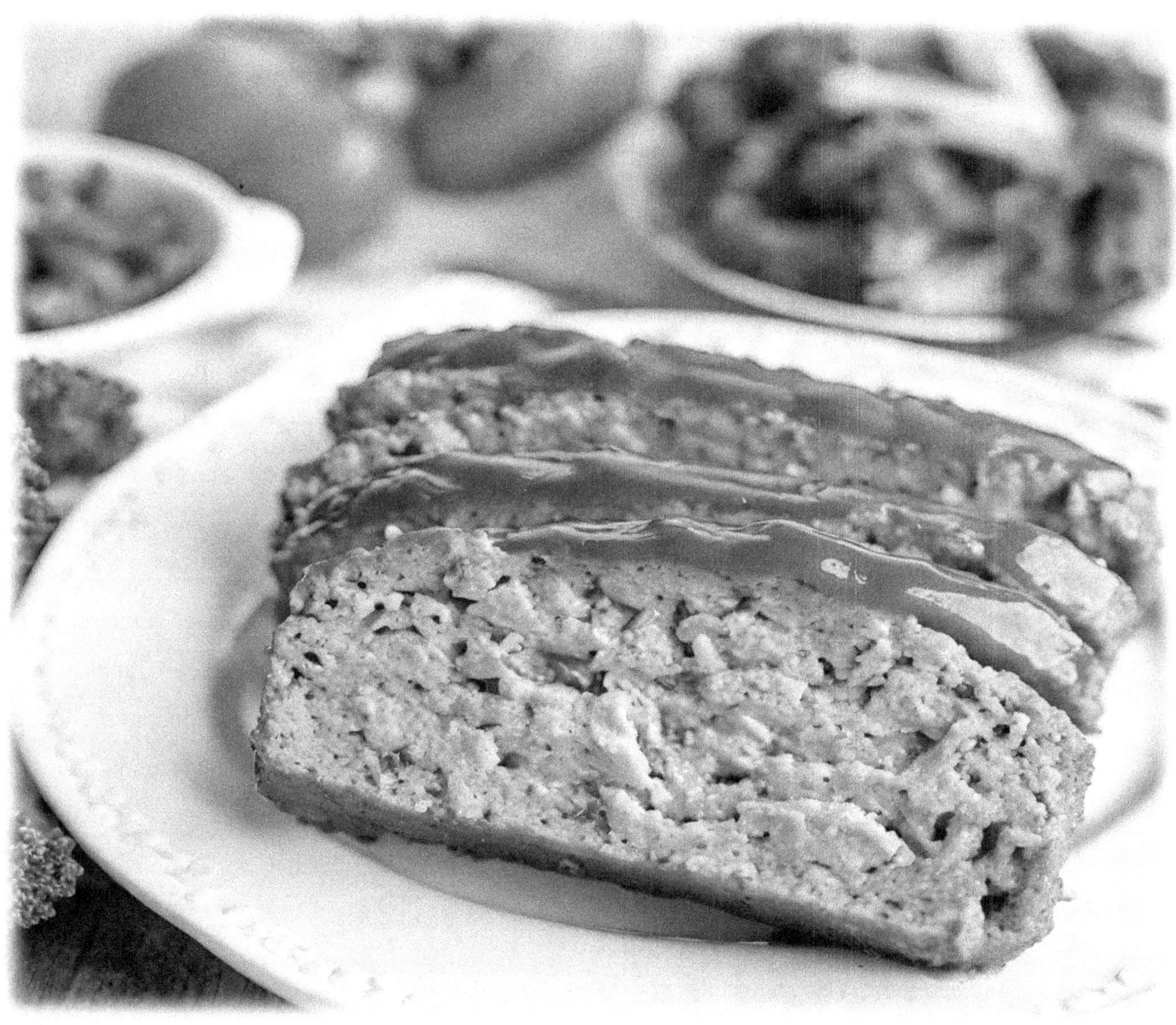

<u>**Nutritional Information:**</u> *Calories: 340.4cal, Protein: 38.8g, Fat: 17.1g, Fiber: 2.4g, Net Carbs: 2.9g*

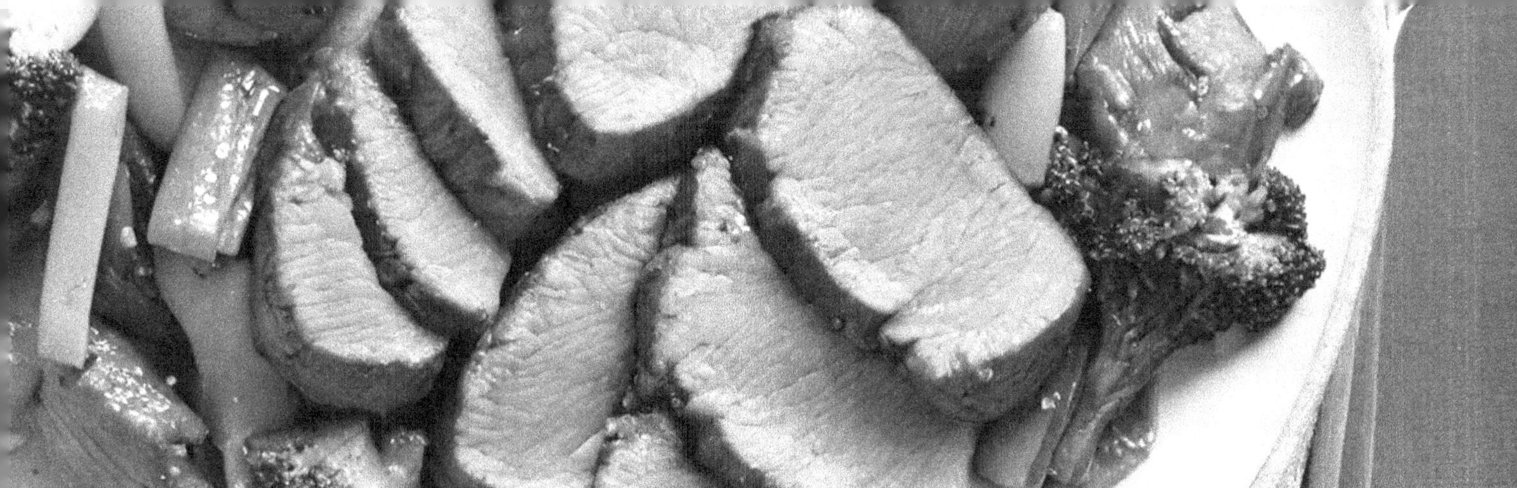

Beef Tenderloin & Vegetable Stir Fry

SERVINGS: 4   PREP TIME: 30 MINUTES   COOK TIME: 15 MINUTES

- 2 pounds of Tenderloin Beef
- 4 ounces of Snow Peas
- 16 ounces of Broccoli Florets
- 1 Red Bell Pepper
- ½ teaspoon of Himalayan Salt
- 1 Large Organic Egg
- 1 ½ teaspoons of Cornstarch
- 1 tablespoon of Low Sodium Soy Sauce
- 2 teaspoons of Black Pepper
- 1 teaspoon of Garlic Powder
- ¼ cup of Cooking Oil
- 1 cup of Low Sodium Soy Sauce
- ¼ cup of Hoison Sauce (you can also use Oyster sauce)
- 1 tablespoon of Shaoxing Cooking Wine (Chinese)
- 2 teaspoons of Pure Sesame Oil

1. Thinly slice the beef tenderloin and remove the excess fat.
2. Add the sliced beef into a large bowl along with the beef marinade ingredients and allow to marinate for at least 30 minutes in the refrigerator.
3. Once your beef is ready, cook your beef for 2 to 3 minutes in a wok, pan or cast iron skillet.
4. Slice your red bell peppers into strips and sautée them along with the broccoli in a half cup of water for 5 minutes at a high-heat.
5. Add the snow peas to the pan and cook them along with the other vegetables for an additional 5 minutes.

- 2 tablespoons of Light Brown Sugar

- 1 teaspoon of Lemon Juice

- 2 teaspoons of Water

- ½ teaspoon of Ground Ginger

- ¼ teaspoon of Ground Cumin

- ¼ teaspoon of Red Cayenne Pepper (optional)

Tips for Variation:

- You can use other tender cuts of beef including sirloin, ribeye, strip loin, or flat iron.

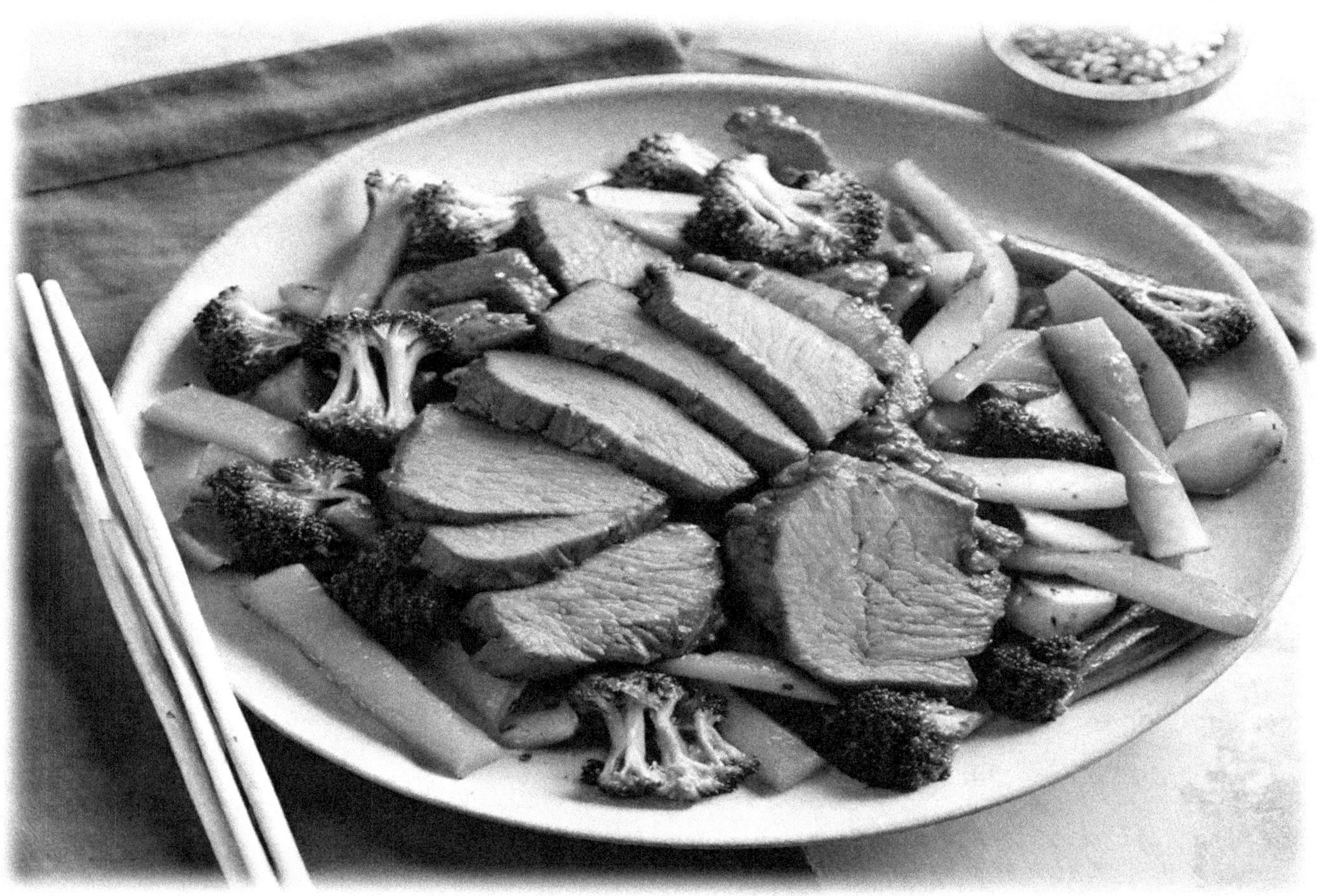

<u>**Nutritional Information:**</u> *Calories: 320 kcal, Total Fat: 25g, Saturated Fat: 7g, Cholesterol: 375mg, Sodium: 400mg, Total Carbohydrates: 5g, Dietary Fiber: 3g, Sugars: 0g, Protein: 20g*

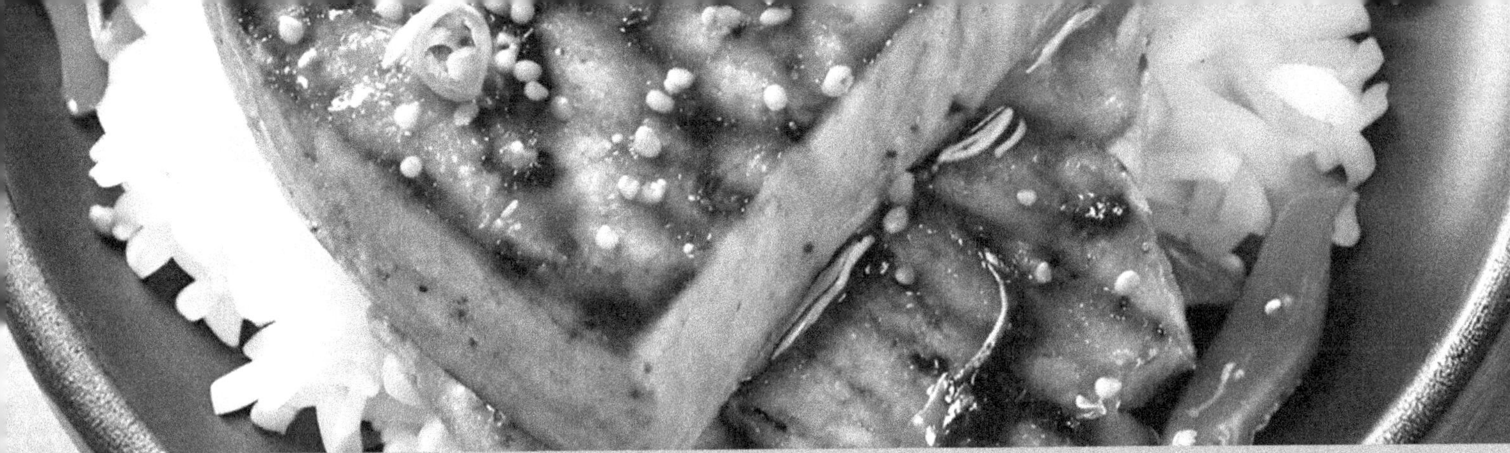

Spicy Tofu Steak

SERVINGS: 2   PREP TIME: 5 MINUTES   COOK TIME: 10 MINUTES

- 1 block (14 oz.) of firm tofu
- 2 tablespoons of olive oil
- 1 tablespoon of soy sauce (low sodium)
- 1 tablespoon of chili powder
- 1 teaspoon of garlic powder
- Salt and pepper to taste

1. Drain the tofu and press it to remove excess water.
2. Cut the tofu into 1/2 inch thick steaks.
3. In a bowl, mix the olive oil, soy sauce, chili powder, and garlic powder.
4. Marinate the tofu steaks in the mixture for at least 30 minutes.
5. Heat a non-stick pan over medium heat.
6. Cook the tofu steaks for about 5 minutes on each side or until they are golden brown.
7. Season with salt and pepper to taste.

<u>Tips for Variation:</u>
- You can add other spices like cumin or paprika to the marinade for different flavors.
- Try grilling the tofu steaks for a smoky flavor.
- Serve with a side of low-carb vegetables like broccoli or spinach for a complete meal.

<u>**Nutritional Information:**</u> *Calories: 200, Protein: 12g, Fat: 15g, Carbohydrates: 5g, Fiber: 2g, Net Carbs: 3g*

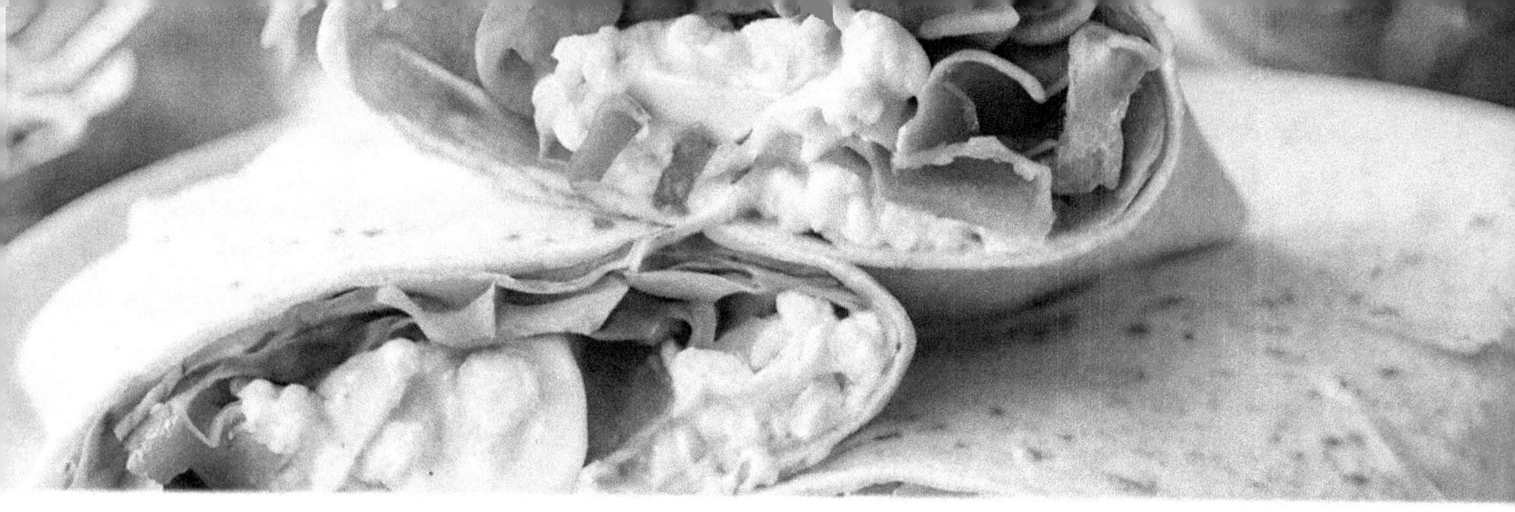

Bacon-Egg Salad Flatout Wrap

SERVINGS: 2   PREP TIME: 15 MINUTES   COOK TIME: 0 MINUTES

INGREDIENTS

- 2 Flatout wraps
- 4 slices of cooked bacon
- 2 hard-boiled eggs
- 1/4 cup of mayonnaise
- Salt and pepper to taste
- 1/2 cup of lettuce
- 1/4 cup of diced tomatoes

INSTRUCTIONS

1. Chop the hard-boiled eggs and cooked bacon into small pieces.
2. In a bowl, mix the chopped eggs, bacon, and mayonnaise. Season with salt and pepper to taste.
3. Lay out the Flatout wraps and evenly distribute the lettuce and diced tomatoes.
4. Spread the egg and bacon mixture on top of the vegetables.
5. Roll up the wraps and cut in half before serving.

Tips for Variation:

- You can add other vegetables like cucumber or bell peppers for extra crunch and flavor.
- Try using turkey bacon for a lower-fat option.
- For a different flavor, you can use flavored mayonnaise or add spices to the egg and bacon mixture.

Nutritional Information: *Calories: 350, Protein: 15g, Fat: 25g, Carbohydrates: 15g, Fiber: 9g, Net Carbs: 6g*

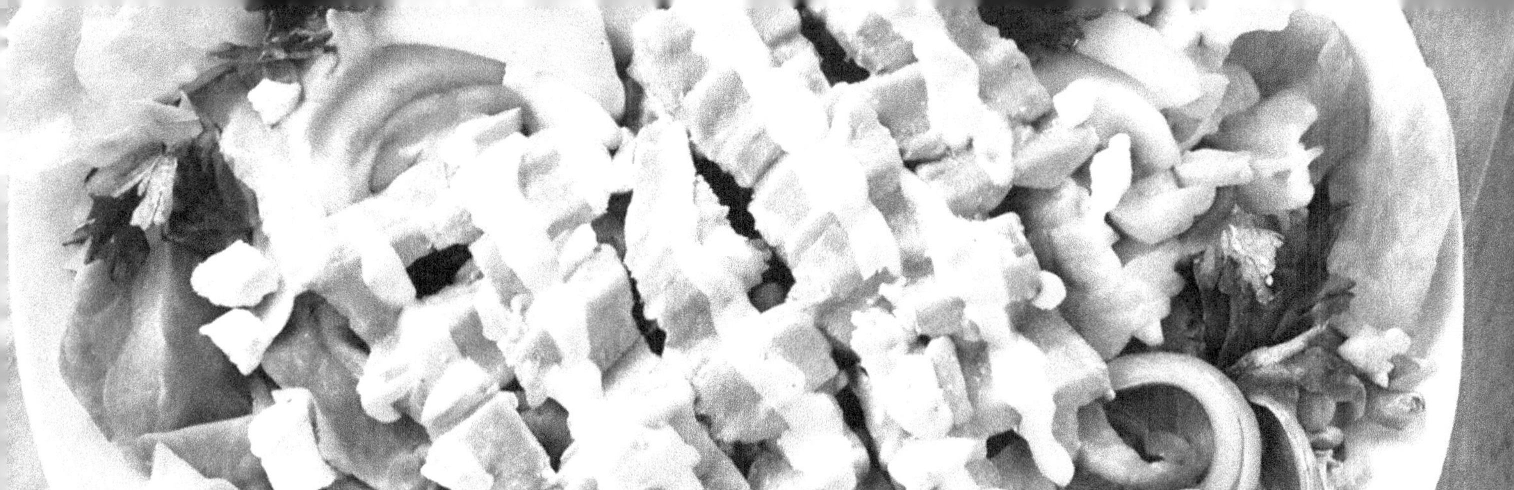

Buffalo Chicken Salad

- 2 boneless, skinless chicken breasts
- 1/4 cup of buffalo sauce
- 4 cups of mixed salad greens
- 1/2 cup of diced celery
- 1/4 cup of diced red onion
- 1/4 cup of blue cheese crumbles
- 2 tablespoons of ranch dressing

1. Cook the chicken breasts in a pan over medium heat until they are no longer pink in the center.
2. Let the chicken cool, then cut it into bite-sized pieces.
3. Toss the chicken pieces in the buffalo sauce.
4. Arrange the salad greens on two plates.
5. Top the greens with the buffalo chicken, celery, red onion, and blue cheese crumbles.
6. Drizzle the ranch dressing over the top of each salad.

Tips for Variation:

- You can add other vegetables like cucumber or bell peppers for extra crunch.
- Try using grilled chicken for a smoky flavor.
- For a different flavor, you can use a different type of cheese like feta or goat cheese.

Nutritional Information: *Calories: 350, Protein: 30g, Fat: 20g, Carbohydrates: 10g, Fiber: 3g, Net Carbs: 7g*

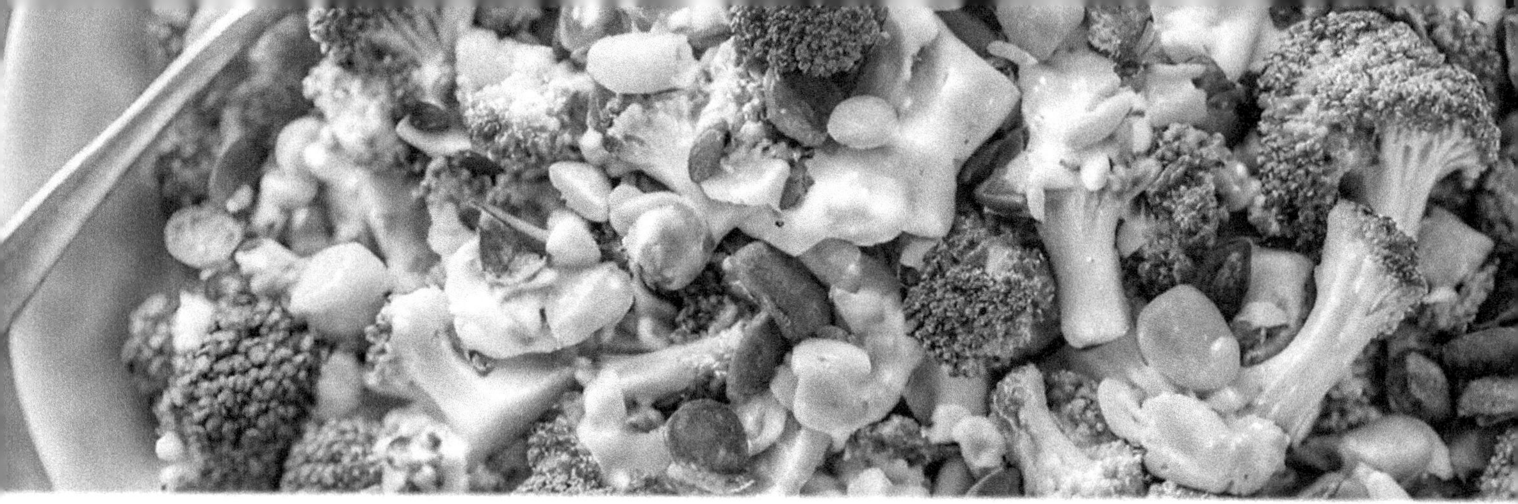

Loaded Broccoli Salad

SERVINGS: 4   PREP TIME: 15 MINUTES   COOK TIME: 0 MINUTES

INGREDIENTS

- 4 cups of broccoli florets
- 1/2 cup of shredded cheddar cheese
- 1/4 cup of diced red onion
- 1/4 cup of sunflower seeds
- 4 slices of cooked bacon, crumbled
- 1/2 cup of mayonnaise
- 1 tablespoon of apple cider vinegar
- Salt and pepper to taste

INSTRUCTIONS

1. In a large bowl, combine the broccoli, cheddar cheese, red onion, sunflower seeds, and crumbled bacon.
2. In a small bowl, whisk together the mayonnaise and apple cider vinegar. Season with salt and pepper to taste.
3. Pour the dressing over the broccoli mixture and toss to coat.
4. Refrigerate for at least 1 hour before serving to allow the flavors to meld together.

Tips for Variation:

- You can add other vegetables like cucumber or bell peppers for extra crunch and flavor.
- Try using turkey bacon for a lower-fat option.
- For a different flavor, you can use flavored mayonnaise or add spices to the egg and bacon mixture.

Nutritional Information: *Calories: 350, Protein: 15g, Fat: 25g, Carbohydrates: 15g, Fiber: 9g, Net Carbs: 6g*

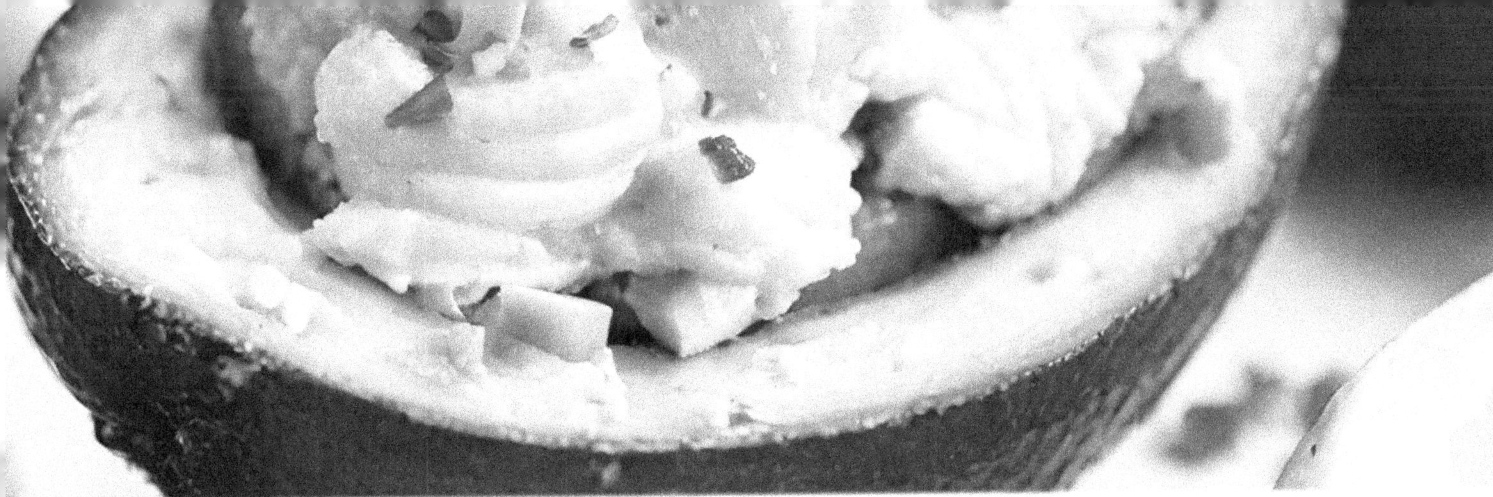

Salmon-Stuffed Avocados

- 2 ripe avocados
- 1 can (6 oz.) of salmon, drained
- 2 tablespoons of mayonnaise
- 1 tablespoon of lemon juice
- Salt and pepper to taste
- 2 tablespoons of chopped fresh dill

1. Cut the avocados in half and remove the pits.
2. In a bowl, mix the salmon, mayonnaise, lemon juice, salt, pepper, and dill.
3. Spoon the salmon mixture into the avocado halves.
4. Serve immediately or refrigerate until ready to serve.

Tips for Variation:

- You can add other ingredients like diced cucumber or bell peppers for extra crunch.
- Try using smoked salmon for a different flavor.
- For a creamier texture, you can add a tablespoon of Greek yogurt to the salmon mixture.

Nutritional Information: *Calories: 250, Protein: 10g, Fat: 20g, Carbohydrates: 10g, Fiber: 7g, Net Carbs: 3g*

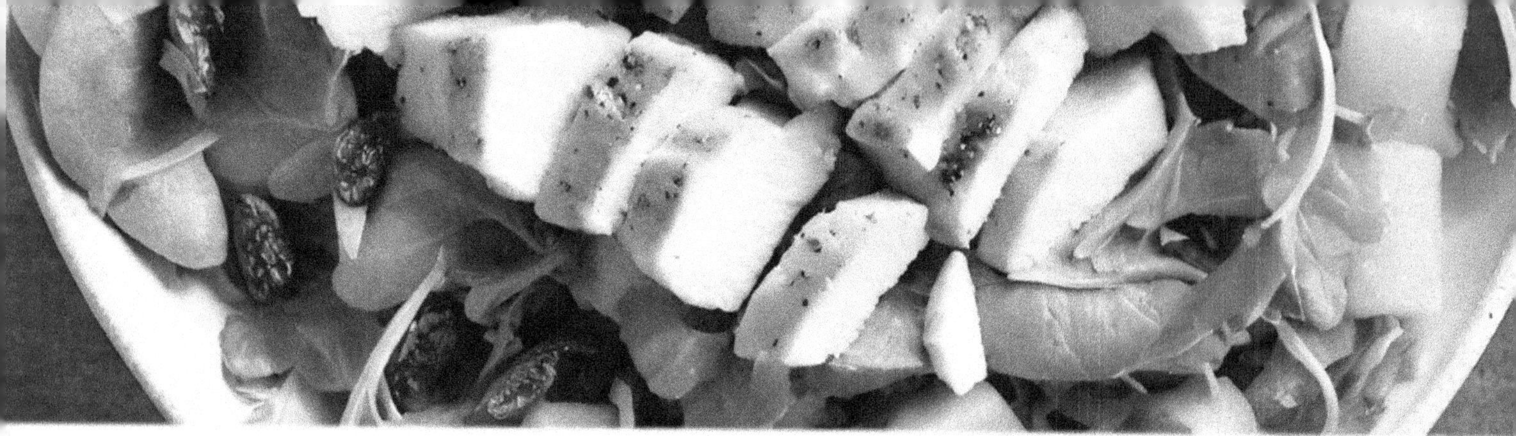

Arugula, Chicken & Melon Salad with Sumac Dressing

SERVINGS: 2   PREP TIME: 10 MINUTES   COOK TIME: 15 MINUTES

INGREDIENTS

- 2 cups of arugula
- 1 cup of cooked chicken breast, sliced
- 1 cup of melon, cubed
- 2 tablespoons of olive oil
- 1 tablespoon of lemon juice
- 1 teaspoon of sumac
- Salt and pepper to taste

INSTRUCTIONS

1. In a large bowl, combine the arugula, chicken, and melon.
2. In a small bowl, whisk together the olive oil, lemon juice, sumac, salt, and pepper to make the dressing.
3. Drizzle the dressing over the salad and toss to combine.
4. Serve immediately or refrigerate until ready to serve.

Tips for Variation:

- You can add other fruits like berries or peaches for a different flavor.
- Try using grilled chicken for a smoky flavor.
- For a different flavor, you can use a different type of greens like spinach or kale.

Nutritional Information: *Calories: 250, Protein: 20g, Fat: 15g, Carbohydrates: 10g, Fiber: 2g, Net Carbs: 8g*

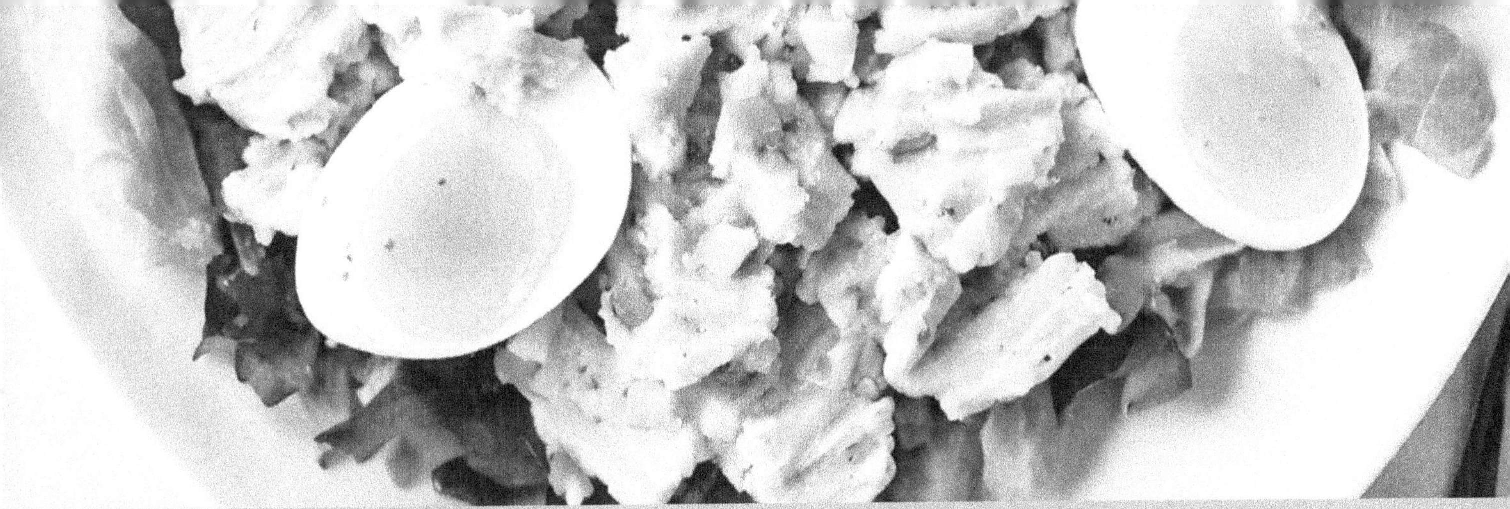

Tuna Salad with Egg

SERVINGS: 2   PREP TIME: 10 MINUTES   COOK TIME: 0 MINUTE

- 1 can (5 oz.) of tuna, drained
- 2 hard-boiled eggs, chopped
- 1/4 cup of mayonnaise
- 1 tablespoon of lemon juice
- 1 teaspoon of sumac
- Salt and pepper to taste
- 2 cups of mixed salad greens

1. In a bowl, mix the tuna, chopped eggs, mayonnaise, lemon juice, sumac, salt, and pepper.
2. Arrange the salad greens on two plates.
3. Top the greens with the tuna and egg mixture.
4. Serve immediately or refrigerate until ready to serve.

Tips for Variation:
- You can add other vegetables like cucumber or bell peppers for extra crunch.
- Try using smoked salmon instead of tuna for a different flavor.
- For a creamier texture, you can add a tablespoon of Greek yogurt to the tuna and egg mixture.

Nutritional Information: *Calories: 300, Protein: 25g, Fat: 20g, Carbohydrates: 5g, Fiber: 2g, Net Carbs: 3g*

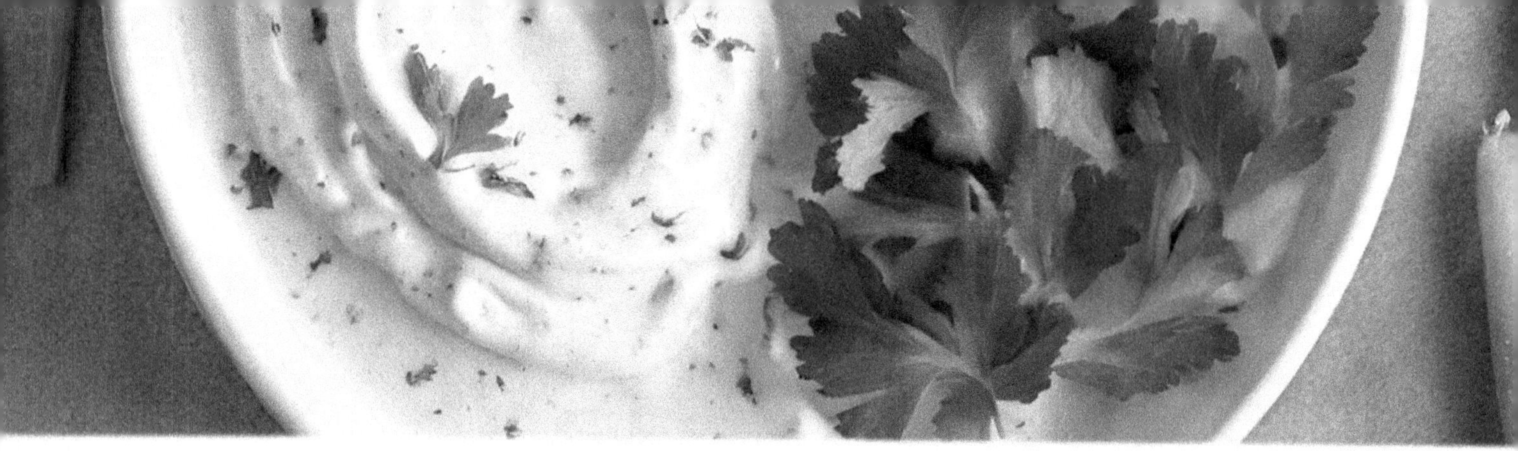

Garlic Ranch Dip with Sumac Dressing

SERVINGS: 8   PREP TIME: 10 MINUTES   COOK TIME: 0 MINUTES

INGREDIENTS

- 1 cup of sour cream
- 1/2 cup of mayonnaise
- 1 tablespoon of ranch seasoning mix
- 2 cloves of garlic, minced
- 1 tablespoon of lemon juice
- 1 teaspoon of sumac
- Salt and pepper to taste

INSTRUCTIONS

1. In a bowl, combine the sour cream, mayonnaise, ranch seasoning mix, minced garlic, lemon juice, sumac, salt, and pepper.
2. Stir until all the ingredients are well combined.
3. Cover the bowl and refrigerate for at least 1 hour before serving to allow the flavors to meld together.
4. Serve with a variety of low-carb vegetables like cucumber slices, bell pepper strips, and celery sticks.

<u>Tips for Variation:</u>

- You can add other spices like paprika or cayenne pepper for a kick.
- Try using Greek yogurt instead of sour cream for a lower-fat option.
- For a different flavor, you can add fresh herbs like dill or parsley.

<u>Nutritional Information:</u> *Calories: 150, Protein: 1g, Fat: 15g, Carbohydrates: 2g, Fiber: 0g, Net Carbs: 2g*

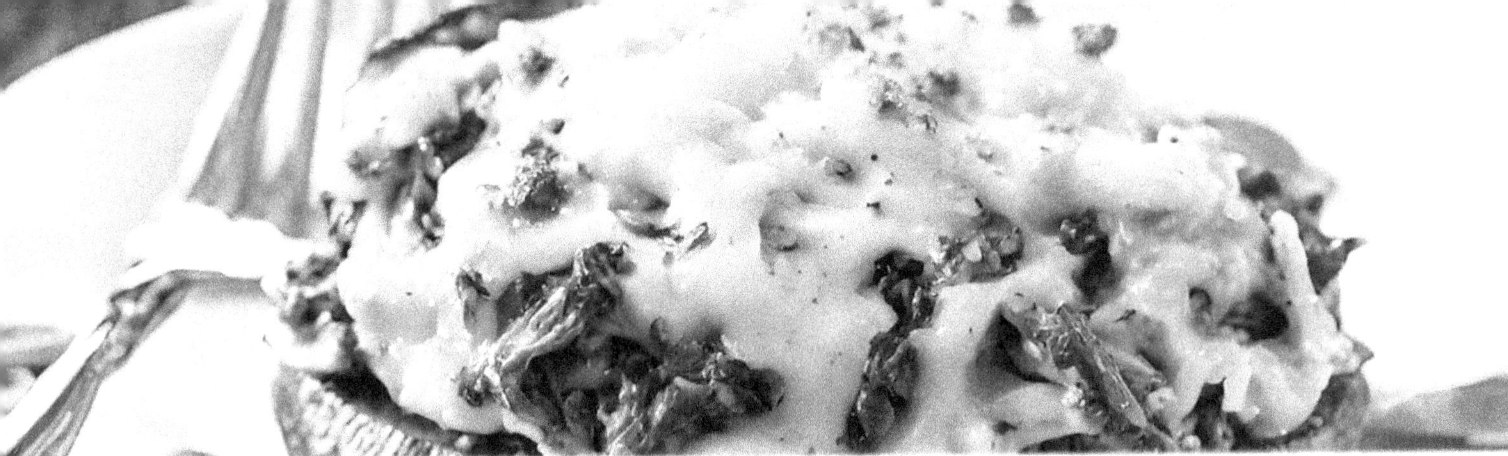

Spinach & Artichoke-Stuffed Portobello Mushrooms

- 4 large portobello mushrooms
- 1 cup of spinach, chopped
- 1/2 cup of canned artichoke hearts, drained and chopped
- 1/2 cup of cream cheese
- 1/4 cup of grated Parmesan cheese
- 2 cloves of garlic, minced
- Salt and pepper to taste

1. Preheat your oven to 375°F (190°C).
2. Remove the stems from the portobello mushrooms and scoop out the gills.
3. In a bowl, mix the spinach, artichoke hearts, cream cheese, Parmesan cheese, minced garlic, salt, and pepper.
4. Stuff each mushroom cap with the spinach and artichoke mixture.
5. Place the stuffed mushrooms on a baking sheet and bake for 15-20 minutes or until the mushrooms are tender and the filling is heated through.

Tips for Variation:

- You can add other vegetables like bell peppers or onions to the filling for extra flavor.
- Try using different types of cheese like mozzarella or feta for a different flavor.
- For a non-vegetarian option, you can add cooked bacon or chicken to the filling.

Nutritional Information: Calories: 200, Protein: 8g, Fat: 15g, Carbohydrates: 10g, Fiber: 3g, Net Carbs: 7g

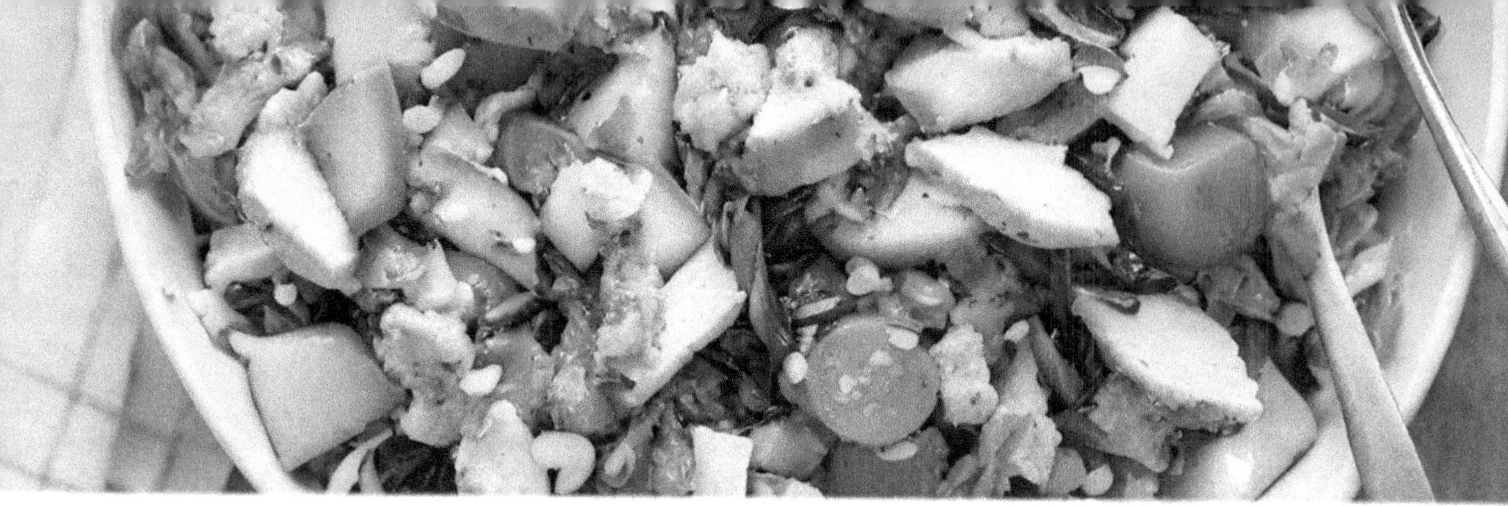

Chopped Power Salad with Chicken

SERVINGS: 4   PREP TIME: 10 MINUTES   COOK TIME: 0 MINUTES

INGREDIENTS

- 2 cups of mixed salad greens
- 1 cup of cooked chicken breast, chopped
- 1/2 cup of cherry tomatoes, halved
- 1/4 cup of cucumber, diced
- 1/4 cup of bell pepper, diced
- 1/4 cup of avocado, diced
- 2 tablespoons of olive oil
- 1 tablespoon of lemon juice
- Salt and pepper to taste

INSTRUCTIONS

1. In a large bowl, combine the salad greens, chicken, cherry tomatoes, cucumber, bell pepper, and avocado.
2. In a small bowl, whisk together the olive oil, lemon juice, salt, and pepper to make the dressing.
3. Drizzle the dressing over the salad and toss to combine.
4. Serve immediately or refrigerate until ready to serve.

Tips for Variation:

- You can add other vegetables like radishes or carrots for extra crunch.
- Try using grilled chicken for a smoky flavor.
- For a different flavor, you can use a different type of dressing like balsamic vinaigrette or ranch dressing.

Nutritional Information: *Calories: 300, Protein: 25g, Fat: 20g, Carbohydrates: 10g, Fiber: 5g, Net Carbs: 5g*

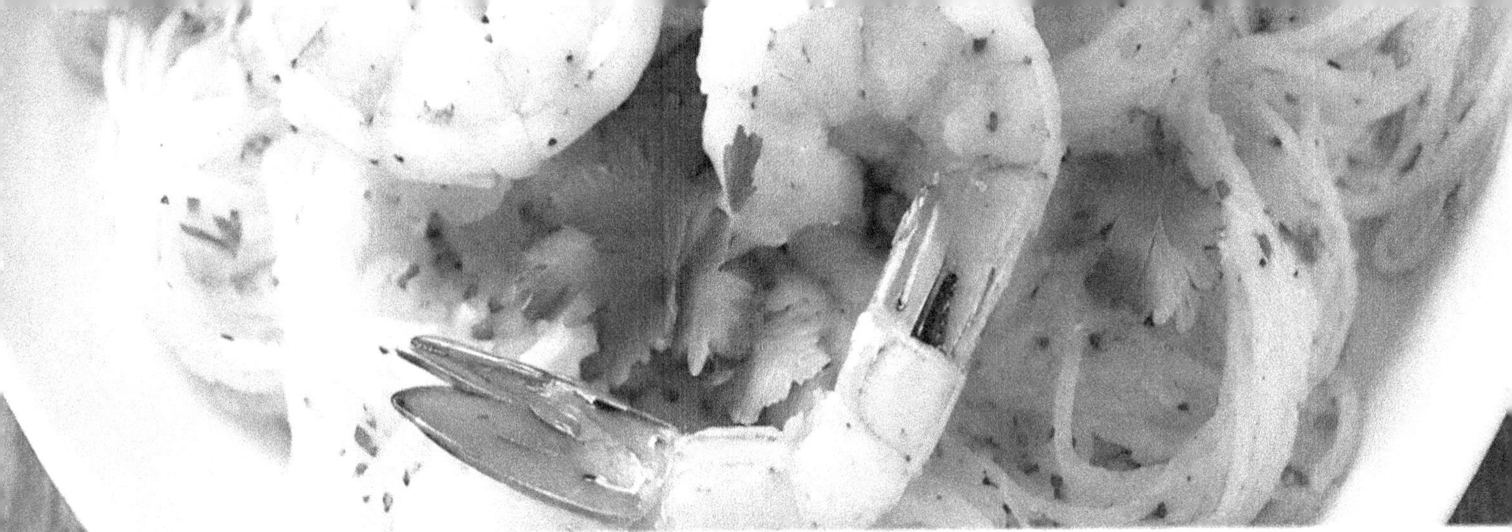

Garlic Shrimp with Cilantro Spaghetti Squash

SERVINGS: 4   PREP TIME: 10 MINUTES   COOK TIME: 50 MINUTES

- 1 medium spaghetti squash
- 1 lb. of shrimp, peeled and deveined
- 4 cloves of garlic, minced
- 2 tablespoons of olive oil
- 1/4 cup of fresh cilantro, chopped
- Salt and pepper to taste

1. Preheat your oven to 400°F (200°C).
2. Cut the spaghetti squash in half lengthwise and scoop out the seeds.
3. Place the squash halves cut-side down on a baking sheet and bake for 40-50 minutes or until the flesh is tender.
4. While the squash is baking, heat the olive oil in a pan over medium heat.
5. Add the minced garlic and cook for 1-2 minutes until fragrant.
6. Add the shrimp to the pan and cook until they are pink and opaque.
7. Season the shrimp with salt and pepper to taste.
8. Once the squash is done, use a fork to scrape out the flesh into spaghetti-like strands.
9. Toss the spaghetti squash strands with the garlic shrimp and chopped cilantro.

Tips for Variation:

- You can add other vegetables like bell peppers or onions for extra flavor.
- Try using grilled chicken instead of shrimp for a different protein source.
- For a different flavor, you can use a different type of herbs like parsley or dill.

Nutritional Information: *Calories: 300, Protein: 25g, Fat: 15g, Carbohydrates: 20g, Fiber: 5g, Net Carbs: 15g*

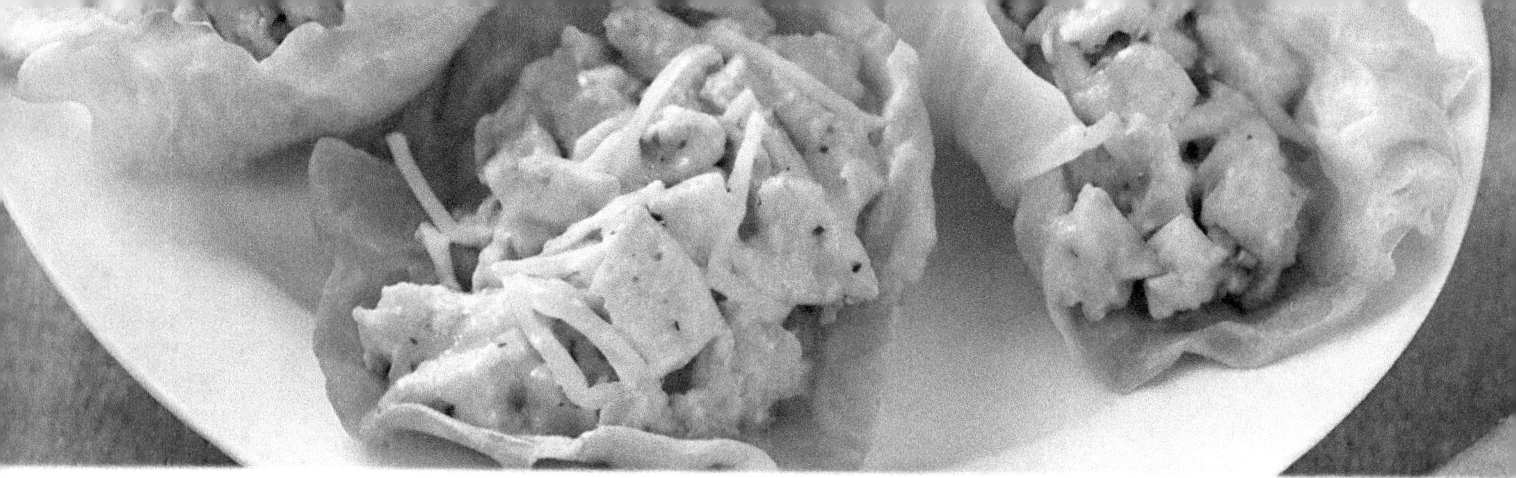

Turkey & Cheddar Lettuce Wraps

SERVINGS: 2   PREP TIME: 10 MINUTES   COOK TIME: 0 MINUTES

INGREDIENTS

- 4 large lettuce leaves
- 1/2 lb. of turkey breast, sliced
- 1/2 cup of cheddar cheese, shredded
- 1/4 cup of mayonnaise
- 1/4 cup of diced tomatoes
- Salt and pepper to taste

INSTRUCTIONS

1. Lay out the lettuce leaves on a flat surface.
2. Spread a tablespoon of mayonnaise on each lettuce leaf.
3. Arrange the turkey slices and shredded cheddar cheese on top of the mayonnaise.
4. Sprinkle the diced tomatoes over the turkey and cheese.
5. Season with salt and pepper to taste.
6. Roll up the lettuce leaves to form the wraps.

Tips for Variation:

- You can add other vegetables like cucumber or bell peppers for extra crunch.
- Try using grilled chicken instead of turkey for a different protein source.
- For a different flavor, you can use a different type of cheese like mozzarella or feta.

Nutritional Information: *Calories: 350, Protein: 30g, Fat: 25g, Carbohydrates: 5g, Fiber: 1g, Net Carbs: 4g*

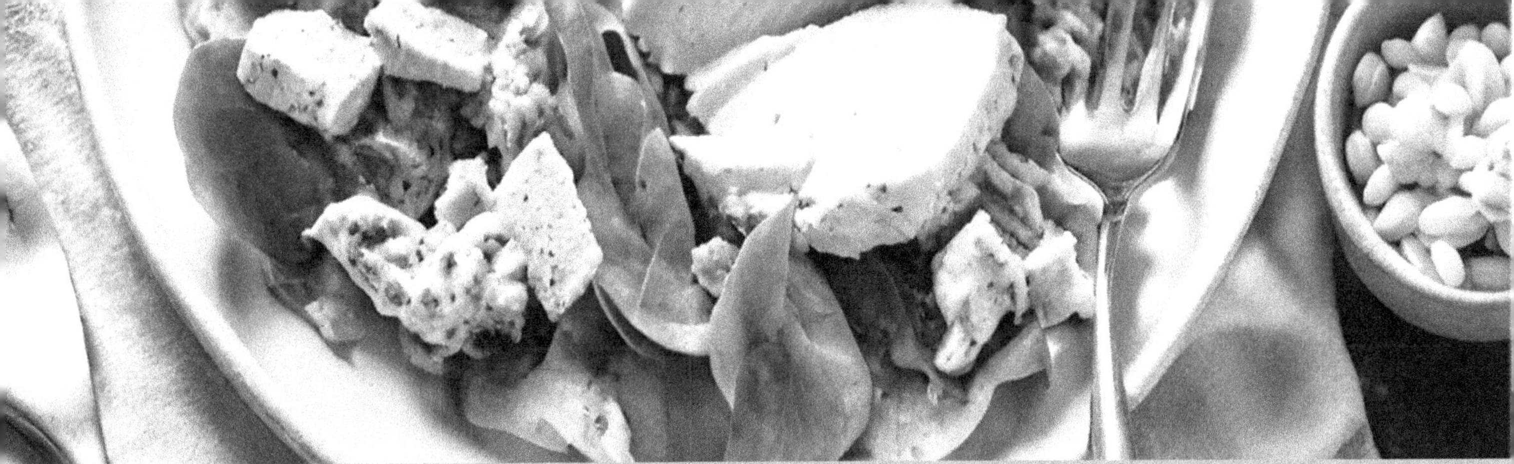

Creamy Pesto Chicken Salad with Greens

SERVINGS: 2   PREP TIME: 10 MINUTES   COOK TIME: 0 MINUTE

- 2 cups of mixed salad greens
- 1 cup of cooked chicken breast, chopped
- 1/4 cup of pesto sauce
- 1/4 cup of mayonnaise
- 1/4 cup of cherry tomatoes, halved
- Salt and pepper to taste

1. In a large bowl, combine the salad greens, chicken, and cherry tomatoes.
2. In a small bowl, mix the pesto sauce and mayonnaise to make the dressing.
3. Drizzle the dressing over the salad and toss to combine.
4. Season with salt and pepper to taste.
5. Serve immediately or refrigerate until ready to serve.

Tips for Variation:
- You can add other vegetables like cucumber or bell peppers for extra crunch.
- Try using grilled chicken for a smoky flavor.
- For a different flavor, you can use a different type of dressing like balsamic vinaigrette or ranch dressing.

Nutritional Information: Calories: 350, Protein: 25g, Fat: 25g, Carbohydrates: 10g, Fiber: 3g, Net Carbs: 7g

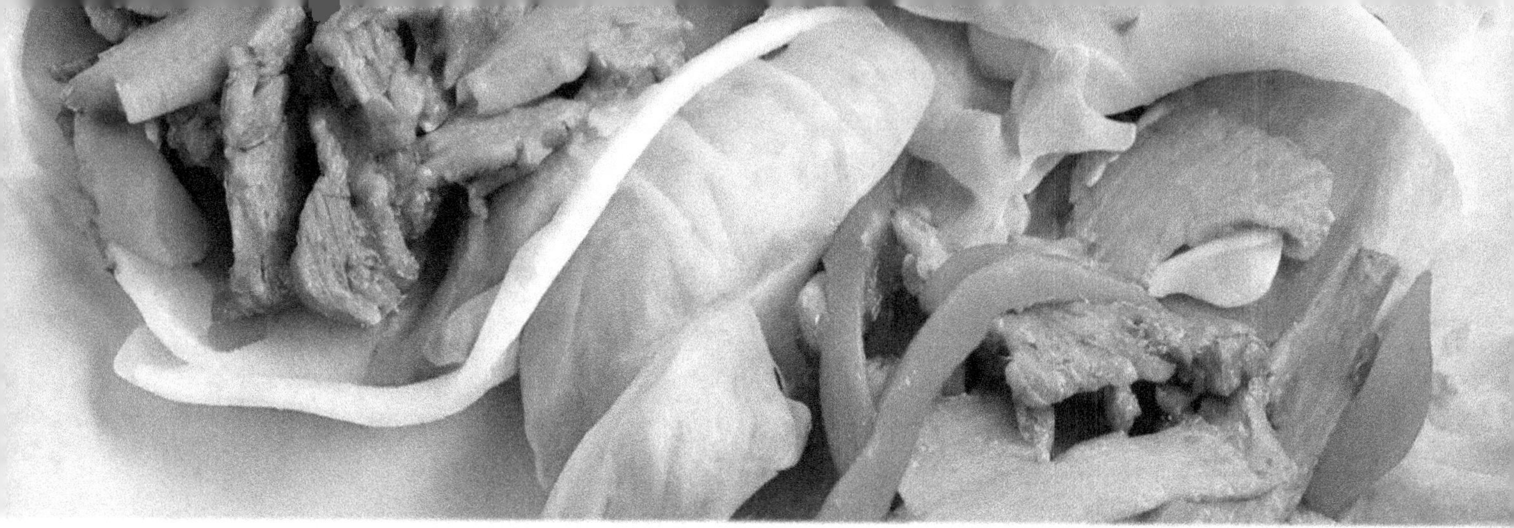

Roast Beef, Red Bell Pepper, and Provolone Lettuce Wraps

INGREDIENTS

- 4 large lettuce leaves
- 1/2 lb. of roast beef, sliced
- 1 red bell pepper, sliced
- 1/2 cup of provolone cheese, sliced
- Salt and pepper to taste

INSTRUCTIONS

1. Lay out the lettuce leaves on a flat surface.
2. Arrange the roast beef, red bell pepper, and provolone cheese on each lettuce leaf.
3. Season with salt and pepper to taste.
4. Roll up the lettuce leaves to form the wraps.

Tips for Variation:

- You can add other vegetables like cucumber or radishes for extra crunch.
- Try using turkey instead of roast beef for a different protein source.
- For a different flavor, you can use a different type of cheese like cheddar or mozzarella.

Nutritional Information: Calories: 350, Protein: 30g, Fat: 20g, Carbohydrates: 10g, Fiber: 3g, Net Carbs: 7g

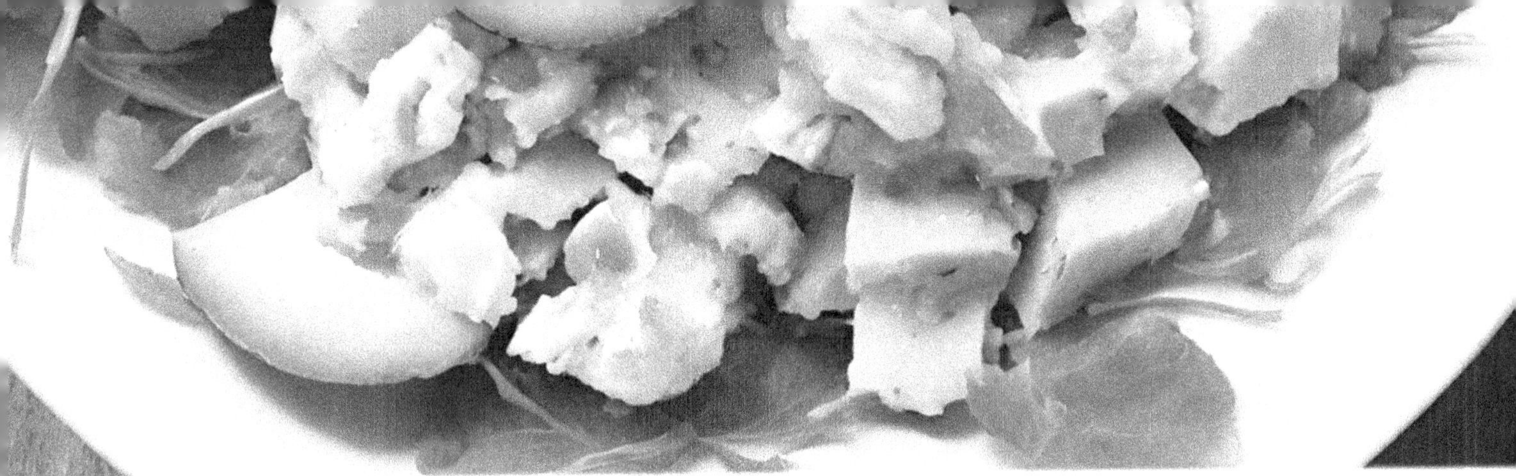

Crab and Avocado Salad

- 1 cup of crab meat
- 1 ripe avocado, diced
- 1/4 cup of diced red onion
- 1/4 cup of diced cucumber
- 2 tablespoons of mayonnaise
- 1 tablespoon of lemon juice
- Salt and pepper to taste
- 2 cups of mixed salad greens

1. In a bowl, combine the crab meat, avocado, red onion, and cucumber.
2. In a small bowl, whisk together the mayonnaise and lemon juice to make the dressing.
3. Pour the dressing over the crab mixture and toss to combine.
4. Season with salt and pepper to taste.
5. Serve the crab and avocado mixture over the salad greens.

Tips for Variation:

- You can add other vegetables like bell peppers or radishes for extra crunch.
- Try using shrimp instead of crab for a different protein source.
- For a different flavor, you can add fresh herbs like dill or parsley.

Nutritional Information: *Calories: 300, Protein: 20g, Fat: 20g, Carbohydrates: 10g, Fiber: 7g, Net Carbs: 3g*

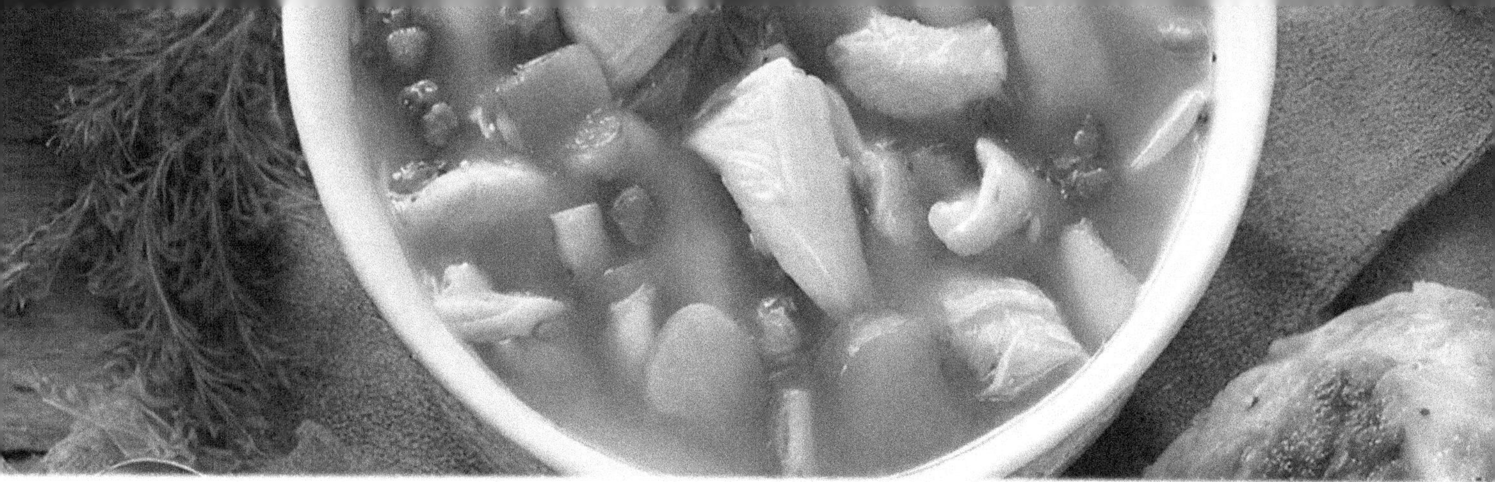

Chicken or Turkey with Vegetable Soup

SERVINGS: 2   PREP TIME: 10 MINUTES   COOK TIME: 30 MINUTES

INGREDIENTS

- 1 lb. of chicken or turkey breast, chopped
- 4 cups of chicken or turkey broth
- 2 cups of mixed vegetables (carrots, celery, bell peppers), chopped
- 1 onion, diced
- 2 cloves of garlic, minced
- 2 tablespoons of olive oil
- Salt and pepper to taste
- 1 teaspoon of dried thyme
- 1 teaspoon of dried rosemary

INSTRUCTIONS

1. Heat the olive oil in a large pot over medium heat.
2. Add the onion and garlic and cook until they are soft and fragrant.
3. Add the chicken or turkey and cook until it is no longer pink.
4. Add the vegetables, broth, salt, pepper, thyme, and rosemary.
5. Bring the soup to a boil, then reduce the heat and let it simmer for 20-30 minutes or until the vegetables are tender.
6. Adjust the seasoning if necessary and serve hot.

Tips for Variation:

- You can add other vegetables like zucchini or spinach for extra nutrients.
- Try using different types of herbs like basil or parsley for a different flavor.
- For a heartier soup, you can add some low-carb noodles or rice.

Nutritional Information: *Calories: 300, Protein: 30g, Fat: 10g, Carbohydrates: 20g, Fiber: 5g, Net Carbs: 15g*

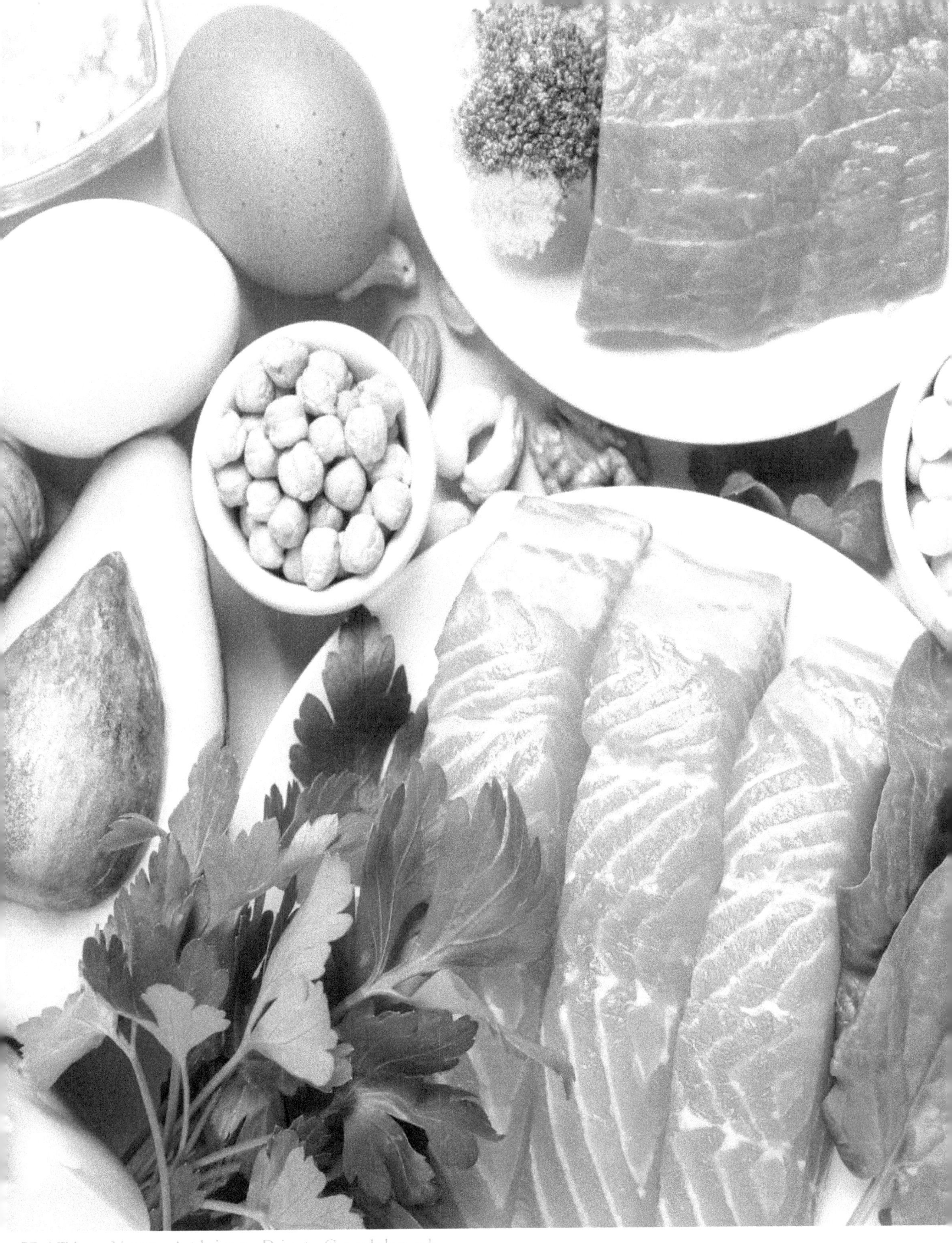

Notes:

Your
Observation:

Progress
Report:

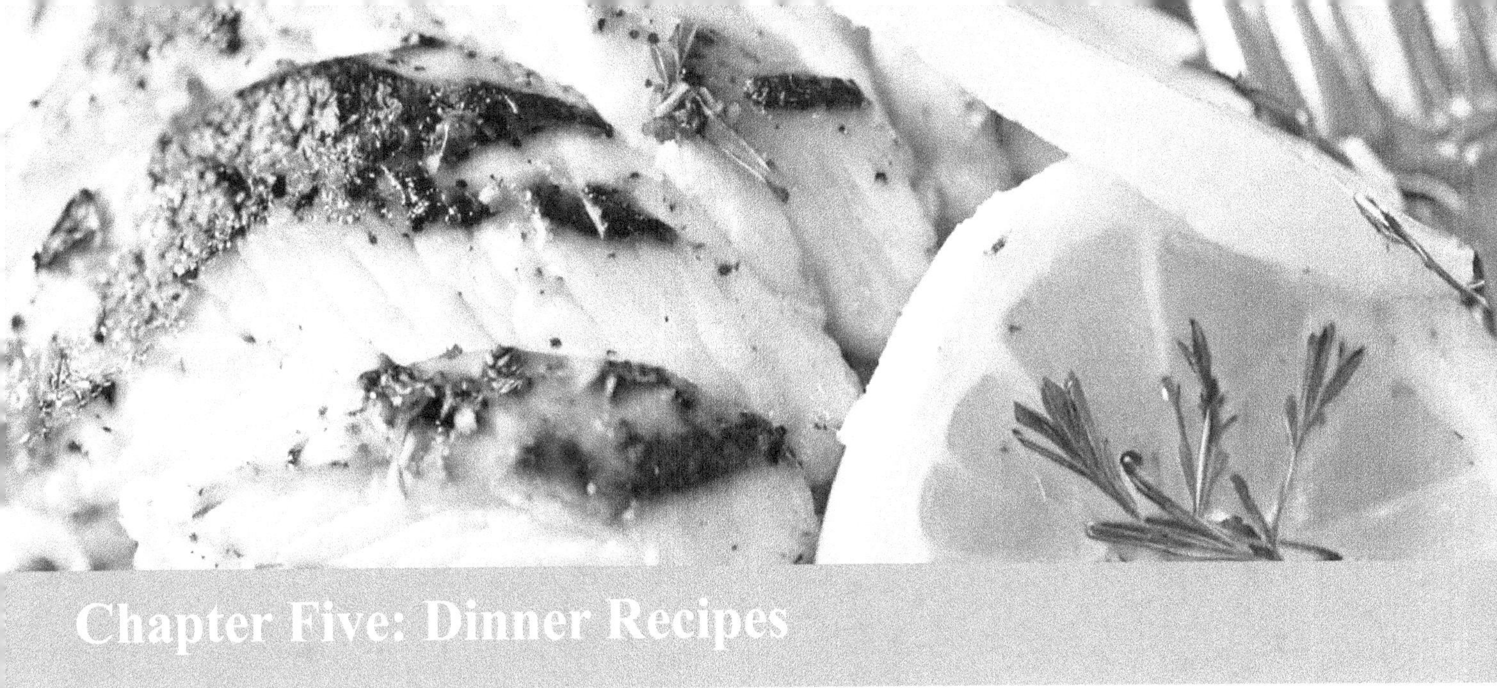

Grilled Lemon Herb Chicken

SERVINGS: 1   PREP TIME: 1 HOUR 10 MINUTES   COOK TIME: 15 MINUTES

INGREDIENTS

- 4 chicken breasts
- 2 lemons, juiced
- 4 cloves of garlic, minced
- 1 tablespoon of fresh rosemary, chopped
- 1 tablespoon of fresh thyme, chopped
- 2 tablespoons of olive oil
- Salt and pepper to taste

INSTRUCTIONS

1. In a bowl, combine the lemon juice, minced garlic, chopped rosemary, chopped thyme, olive oil, salt, and pepper.
2. Add the chicken breasts to the bowl and make sure they are well coated with the marinade.
3. Cover the bowl and let the chicken marinate in the refrigerator for at least 1 hour.
4. Preheat your grill to medium heat.
5. Grill the chicken breasts for 6-7 minutes on each side or until they are no longer pink in the center.

- You can add other herbs like basil or parsley for a different flavor.

- Try using lime juice instead of lemon juice for a tangy twist.

- For a spicier kick, you can add some chili flakes to the marinade.

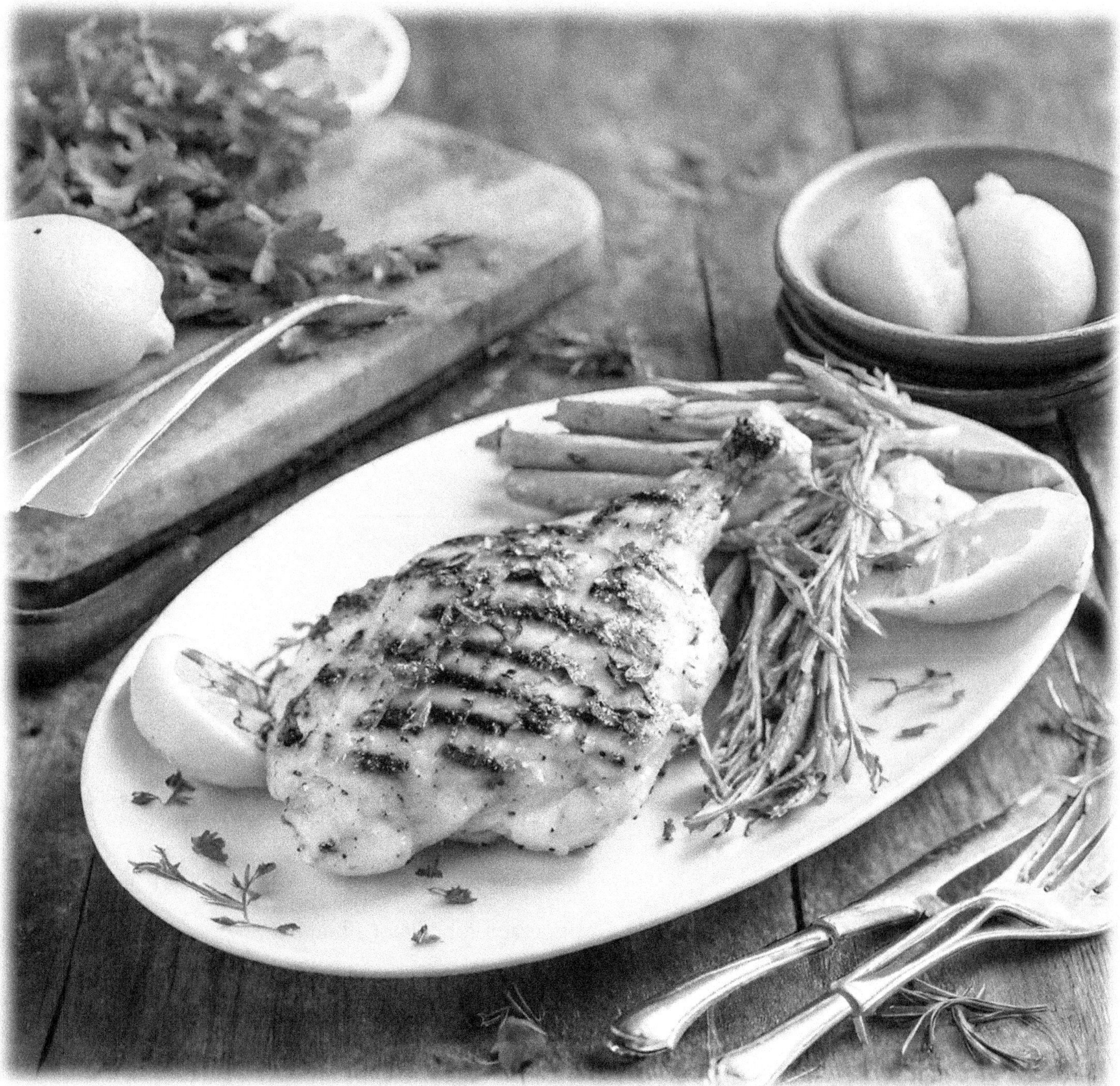

<u>**Nutritional Information (per 3-ounce serving):**</u> *Calories: 300, Protein: 30g, Fat: 15g, Carbohydrates: 5g, Fiber: 1g, Net Carbs: 4g*

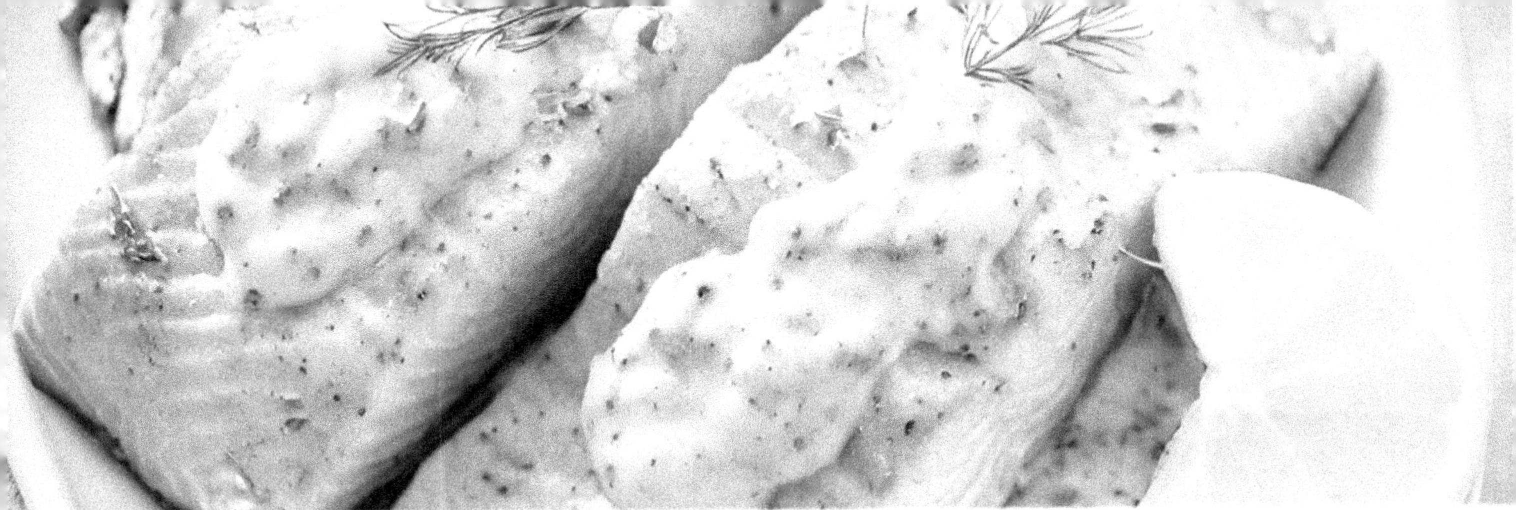

Baked Salmon with Dill Sauce

SERVINGS: 4   PREP TIME: 5 MINUTES   COOK TIME: 15 MINUTES

- 4 salmon fillets
- 2 tablespoons of olive oil
- Salt and pepper to taste
- 1/2 cup of sour cream
- 1 tablespoon of fresh dill, chopped
- 1 tablespoon of lemon juice

1. Preheat your oven to 400°F (200°C).
2. Place the salmon fillets on a baking sheet and drizzle them with olive oil. Season with salt and pepper to taste.
3. Bake the salmon for 12-15 minutes or until it is cooked through.
4. While the salmon is baking, mix the sour cream, chopped dill, and lemon juice in a bowl to make the dill sauce.
5. Serve the baked salmon with the dill sauce on top.

Tips for Variation:

- You can add other herbs like parsley or thyme to the dill sauce for a different flavor.
- Try grilling the salmon for a smoky flavor.
- For a different flavor, you can use a different type of fish like trout or cod.

Nutritional Information: *Calories: 350, Protein: 30g, Fat: 25g, Carbohydrates: 2g, Fiber: 0g, Net Carbs: 2g*

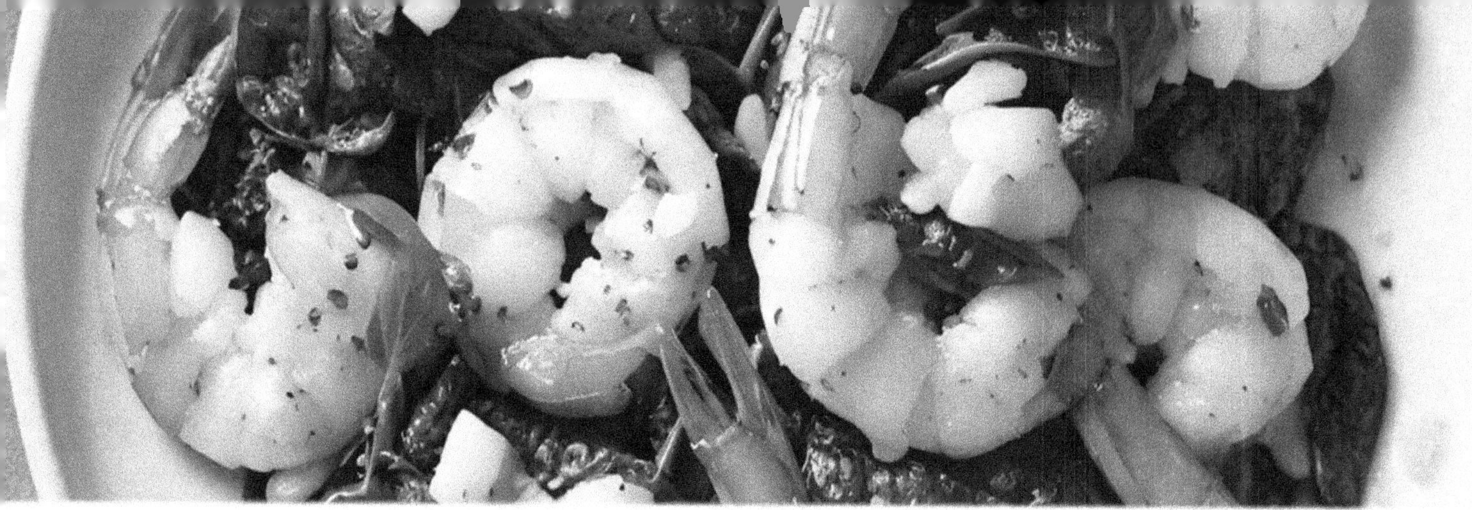

Sautéed Shrimp with Garlic and Spinach

SERVINGS: 4   PREP TIME: 10 MINUTES   COOK TIME: 10 MINUTES

INGREDIENTS

- 1 lb. (450g) shrimp, peeled and deveined
- 2 tablespoons olive oil
- 4 cloves garlic, minced
- 8 cups fresh spinach leaves
- Salt and pepper to taste
- Lemon wedges for serving (optional)

INSTRUCTIONS

1. Heat olive oil in a large skillet over medium heat.
2. Add minced garlic to the skillet and sauté for 1-2 minutes until fragrant.
3. Add shrimp to the skillet and cook for 2-3 minutes on each side until pink and cooked through.
4. Stir in the fresh spinach leaves and cook for an additional 1-2 minutes until wilted.
5. Season with salt and pepper to taste.
6. Serve hot with lemon wedges on the side if desired.

Tips for Variation:

- Add a pinch of red pepper flakes for some heat.
- Sprinkle with grated Parmesan cheese before serving.
- Substitute spinach with other leafy greens like kale or Swiss chard.
- Serve over cauliflower rice or zucchini noodles for a low-carb option.

Nutritional Information: *Calories: 215 kcal, Total Fat: 11g, Saturated Fat: 2g, Cholesterol: 239mg, Sodium: 437mg, Total Carbohydrates: 3g, Dietary Fiber: 2g, Sugars: 0g, Protein: 26g*

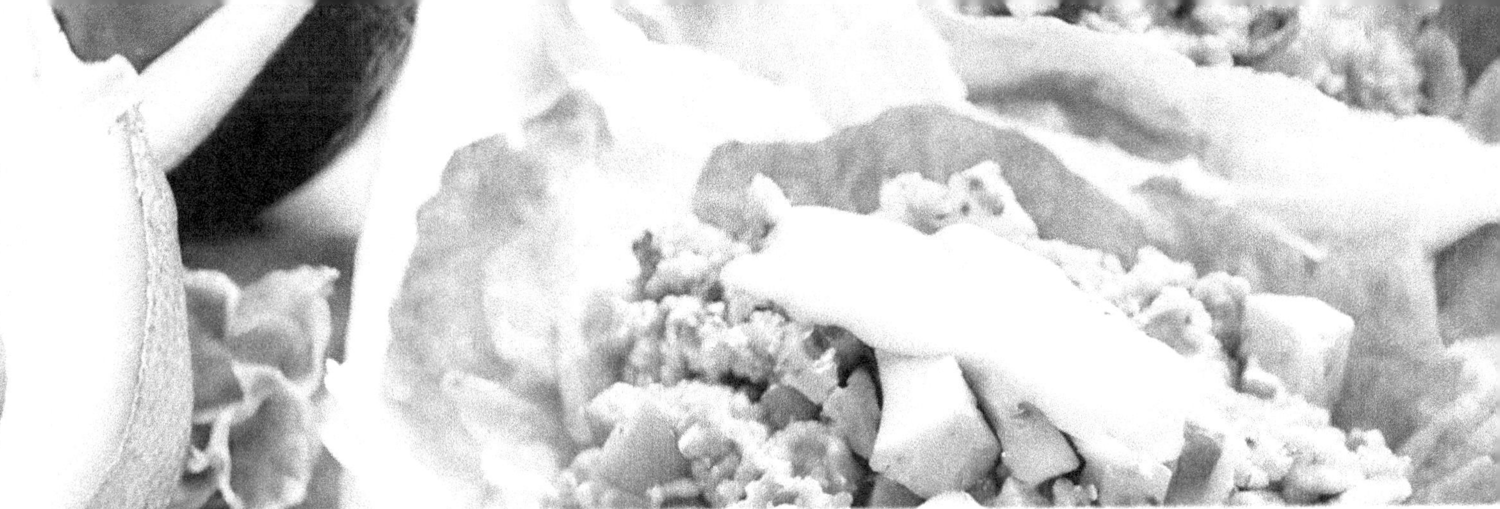

Turkey and Avocado Lettuce Wraps

SERVINGS: 4   PREP TIME: 10 MINUTES   COOK TIME: 10 MINUTES

- 1 lb. (450g) ground turkey
- 2 tablespoons olive oil
- 1 teaspoon garlic powder
- 1 teaspoon onion powder
- Salt and pepper to taste
- 1 large avocado, sliced
- 1 head iceberg or butter lettuce, leaves separated

Tips for Variation:

- Add diced tomatoes, onions, or bell peppers for extra flavor and crunch.
- Substitute ground chicken or beef for the turkey.
- Drizzle with a squeeze of lime juice or your favorite hot sauce for added zest.
- Top with a dollop of Greek yogurt or sour cream for creaminess.

1. Heat olive oil in a skillet over medium heat.
2. Add ground turkey to the skillet and cook, breaking it apart with a spoon, until browned and cooked through, about 5-7 minutes.
3. Season the turkey with garlic powder, onion powder, salt, and pepper, stirring to combine.
4. Remove the skillet from the heat and let the turkey cool slightly.
5. Assemble the lettuce wraps by placing a spoonful of cooked turkey onto each lettuce leaf.
6. Top the turkey with slices of avocado.
7. Roll up the lettuce leaves to form wraps and secure with toothpicks if needed.
8. Serve immediately.

Nutritional Information: Calories: 275 kcal, Total Fat: 17g, Saturated Fat: 3g, Cholesterol: 84mg, Sodium: 83mg, Total, Carbohydrates: 6g, Dietary Fiber: 4g, Sugars: 1g, Protein: 25g

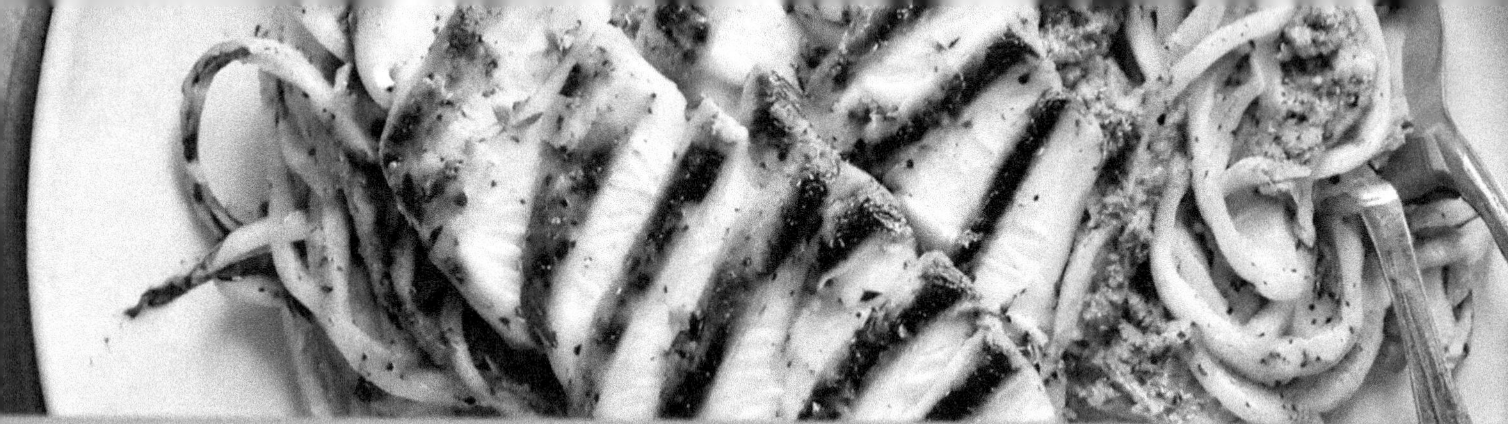

Zucchini Noodles with Pesto and Grilled Chicken

SERVINGS: 2   PREP TIME: 15 MINUTES   COOK TIME: 15 MINUTE

INGREDIENTS

- 2 medium zucchinis
- 2 boneless, skinless chicken breasts
- Salt and pepper to taste
- 2 tablespoons olive oil
- ½ cup homemade or store-bought pesto sauce
- Grated Parmesan cheese for garnish (optional)
- Fresh basil leaves for garnish (optional)

INSTRUCTIONS

1. In a large bowl, combine the salad greens, chicken, and cherry tomatoes.
2. In a small bowl, mix the pesto sauce and mayonnaise to make the dressing.
3. Drizzle the dressing over the salad and toss to combine.
4. Season with salt and pepper to taste.
5. Serve immediately or refrigerate until ready to serve.
6. Add the zucchini noodles to the skillet and sauté for 2-3 minutes, or until just tender.
7. Toss the cooked zucchini noodles with pesto sauce until evenly coated.
8. Divide the zucchini noodles onto serving plates and top with sliced grilled chicken.
9. Garnish with grated Parmesan cheese and fresh basil leaves if desired.
10. Serve immediately.

<u>**Tips for Variation:**</u>

- Use spiralized sweet potatoes or carrots in addition to or instead of zucchini noodles.

- Substitute grilled shrimp or tofu for the chicken for a different protein option.

- Mix in cherry tomatoes or roasted red peppers for added flavor and color.

- Make your own pesto using fresh basil, pine nuts, garlic, Parmesan cheese, and olive oil for a more personalized touch.

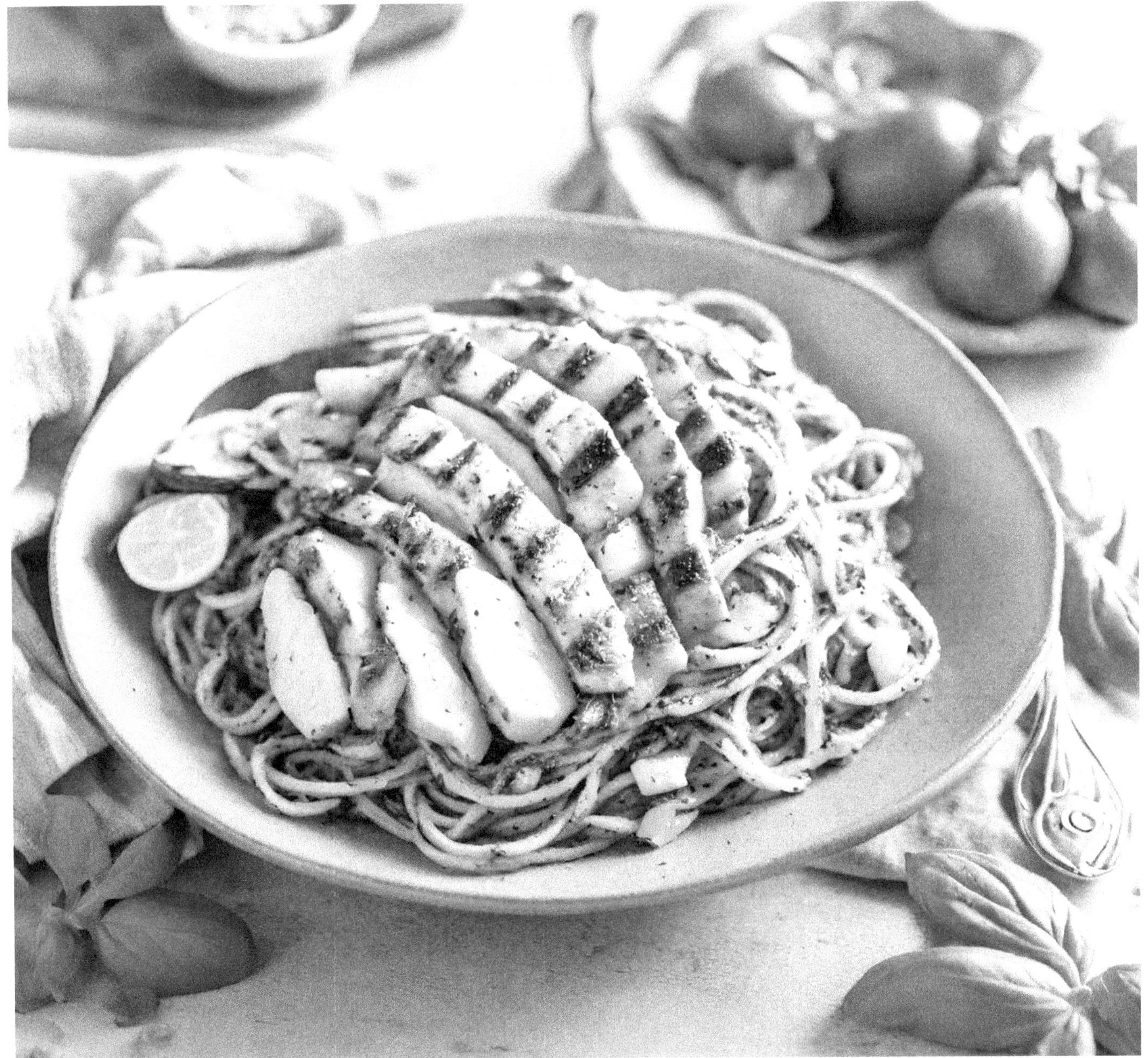

<u>**Nutritional Information:**</u> *Calories: 398 kcal, Total Fat: 25g, Saturated Fat: 4g, Cholesterol: 98mg, Sodium: 424mg, Total Carbohydrates: 7g, Dietary Fiber: 2g, Sugars: 3g, Protein: 36g*

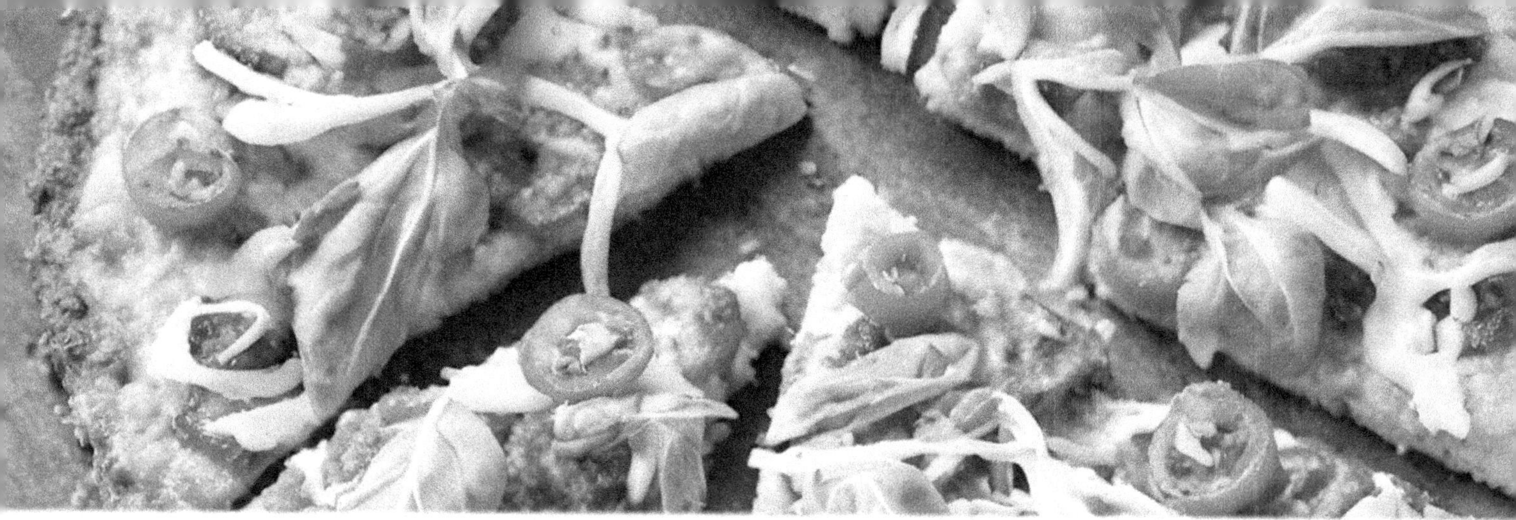

Cauliflower Crust Pizza

SERVINGS: 4   PREP TIME: 20 MINUTES   COOK TIME: 25-30 MINUTES

INGREDIENTS

- 1 medium head cauliflower, riced (about 4 cups)
- 1/2 cup shredded mozzarella cheese
- 1/4 cup grated Parmesan cheese
- 1/2 teaspoon dried oregano
- 1/2 teaspoon garlic powder
- 1/4 teaspoon salt
- 2 eggs
- 1/4 cup almond flour (optional, for added stability)
- Your choice of pizza toppings (e.g., tomato sauce, cheese, vegetables, meats)

INSTRUCTIONS

1. Preheat your oven to 425°F (220°C). Line a baking sheet with parchment paper.
2. Prepare the cauliflower by washing it and cutting it into florets. Place the florets in a food processor and pulse until they resemble rice-like grains.
3. Place the cauliflower rice in a microwave-safe bowl and microwave on high for 4-5 minutes, or until softened. Allow it to cool slightly.
4. Transfer the cooled cauliflower rice to a clean kitchen towel or cheesecloth and wring out as much moisture as possible.
5. In a large mixing bowl, combine the cauliflower rice, shredded mozzarella, grated Parmesan, dried oregano, garlic powder, salt, eggs, and almond flour (if using). Mix until well combined.
6. Spread the cauliflower mixture onto the prepared baking sheet, shaping it into a round pizza crust about 1/4 inch thick.

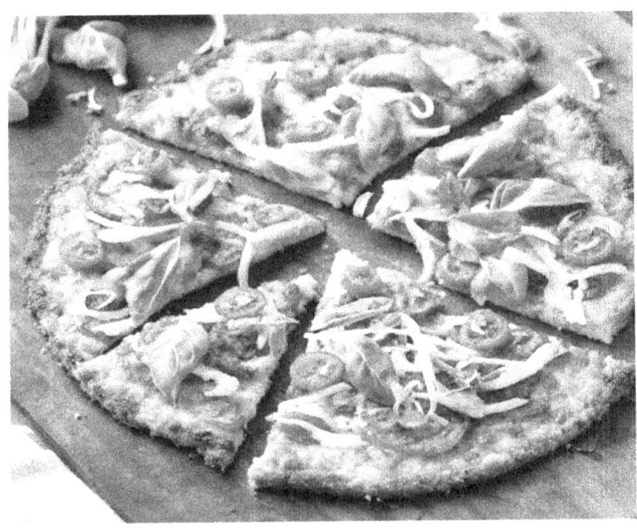

7. Bake the crust in the preheated oven for 15-20 minutes, or until golden brown and firm to the touch.
8. Once the crust is done, remove it from the oven and add your desired pizza toppings.
9. Return the pizza to the oven and bake for an additional 5-10 minutes, or until the cheese is melted and bubbly.
10. Slice and serve hot.

Tips for Variation:

- Experiment with different cheese blends for the crust, such as cheddar, provolone, or goat cheese.
- Customize your pizza toppings to suit your taste preferences and dietary needs. Consider using low-carb options like sugar-free tomato sauce, grilled chicken, spinach, mushrooms, and bell peppers.
- For a crispy crust, bake the cauliflower crust on a pizza stone or pizza pan.
- Make mini pizzas by dividing the cauliflower mixture into smaller portions and shaping them into individual crusts.

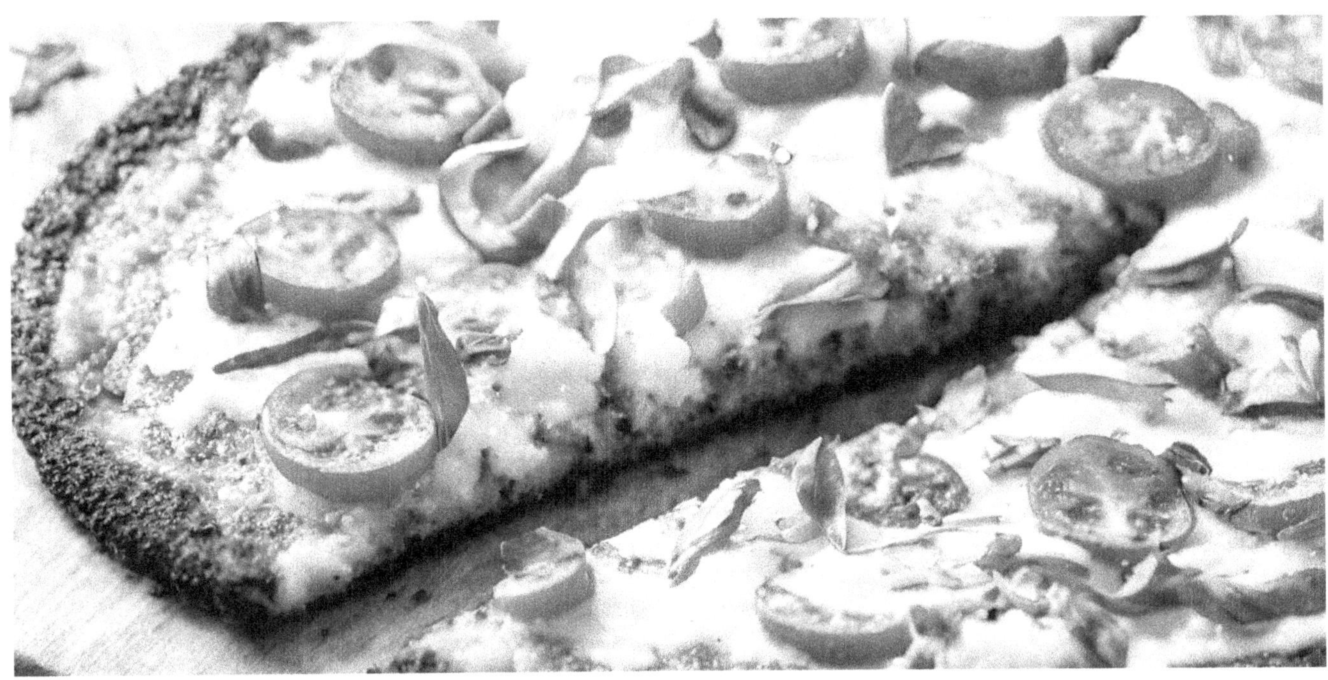

Nutritional Information: *Calories: 135 kcal, Total Fat: 7g, Saturated Fat: 3g, Cholesterol: 74mg, Sodium: 349mg, Total Carbohydrates: 9g, Dietary Fiber: 3g, Sugars: 3g, Protein: 10g*

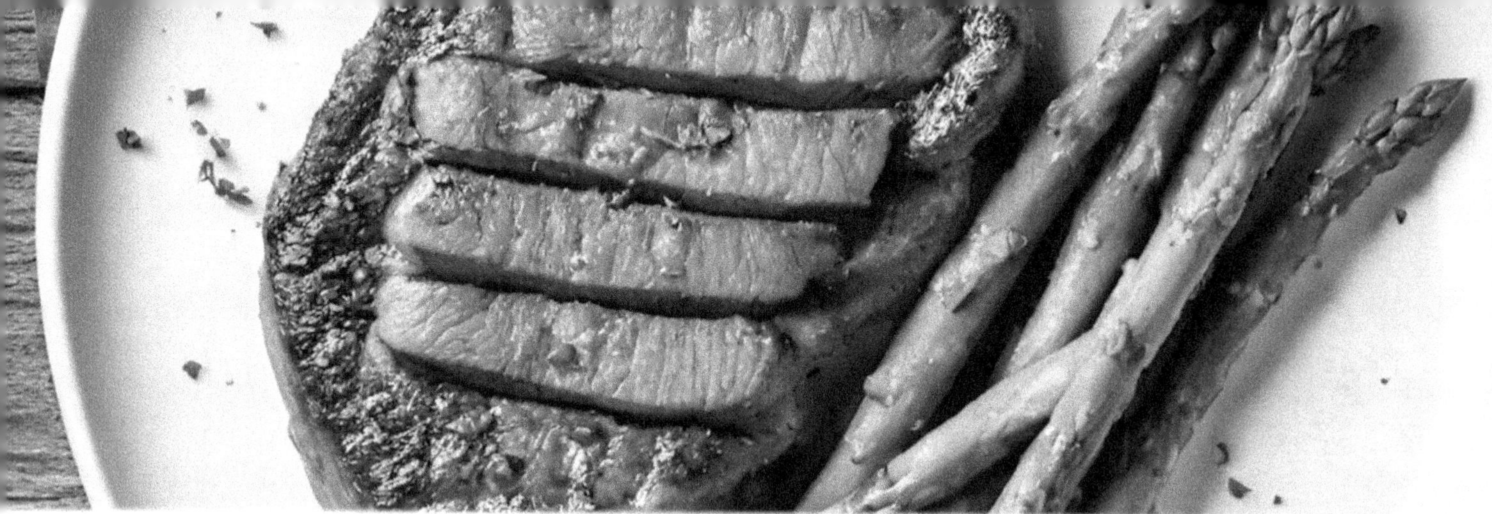

Grilled Steak with Asparagus

INGREDIENTS

- 2 (8-ounce) beef steaks (such as sirloin, ribeye, or filet mignon)
- Salt and pepper to taste
- 1 tablespoon olive oil
- 1 pound fresh asparagus spears, trimmed
- Optional: steak seasoning or marinade of your choice

INSTRUCTIONS

1. Preheat your grill to medium-high heat.
2. Season the steaks generously with salt and pepper on both sides. If desired, you can also use your favorite steak seasoning or marinade.
3. Drizzle olive oil over the asparagus spears and season with salt and pepper.
4. Place the steaks and asparagus on the grill. Cook the steaks to your desired level of doneness, flipping once halfway through. This typically takes about 4-6 minutes per side for medium-rare, depending on the thickness of the steaks.
5. As the steaks cook, grill the asparagus alongside, turning occasionally, until they are tender and slightly charred, about 8-10 minutes.
6. Once the steaks and asparagus are cooked to your liking, remove them from the grill and let the steaks rest for a few minutes before slicing.

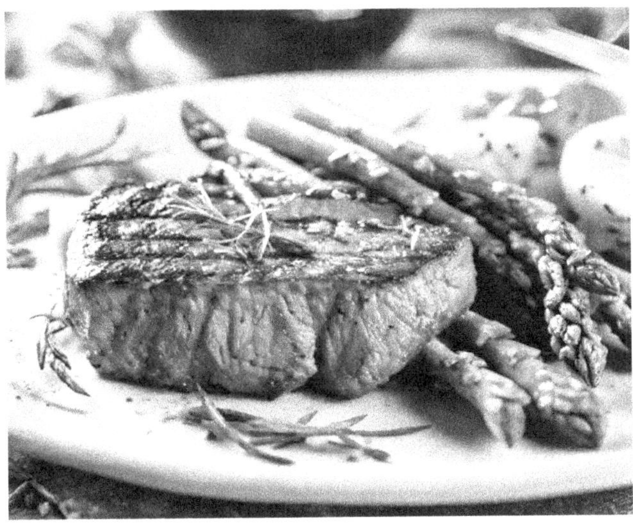

7. Serve the grilled steak slices alongside the grilled asparagus.

<u>Tips for Variation:</u>

- Add minced garlic or chopped fresh herbs (such as rosemary or thyme) to the olive oil for extra flavor.
- Try grilling other vegetables alongside the asparagus, such as bell peppers, zucchini, or cherry tomatoes.
- Serve the steak with a side salad or grilled portobello mushrooms for a low-carb meal option.
- For a different twist, use a dry rub or marinade on the steaks before grilling, such as a spicy Cajun rub or a tangy balsamic marinade.

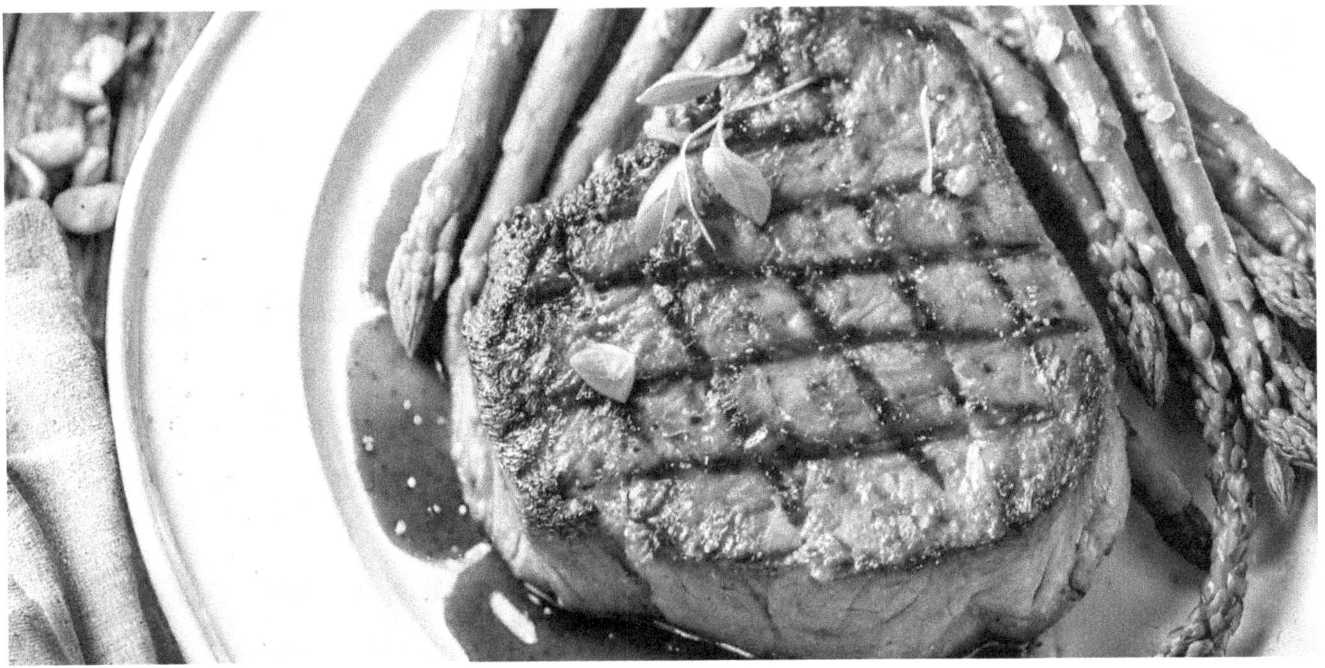

<u>Nutritional Information:</u> *Calories: 400 kcal, Total Fat: 24g, Saturated Fat: 8g, Cholesterol: 120mg, Sodium: 85mg, Total Carbohydrates: 6g, Dietary Fiber: 3g, Sugars: 2g, Protein: 40g*

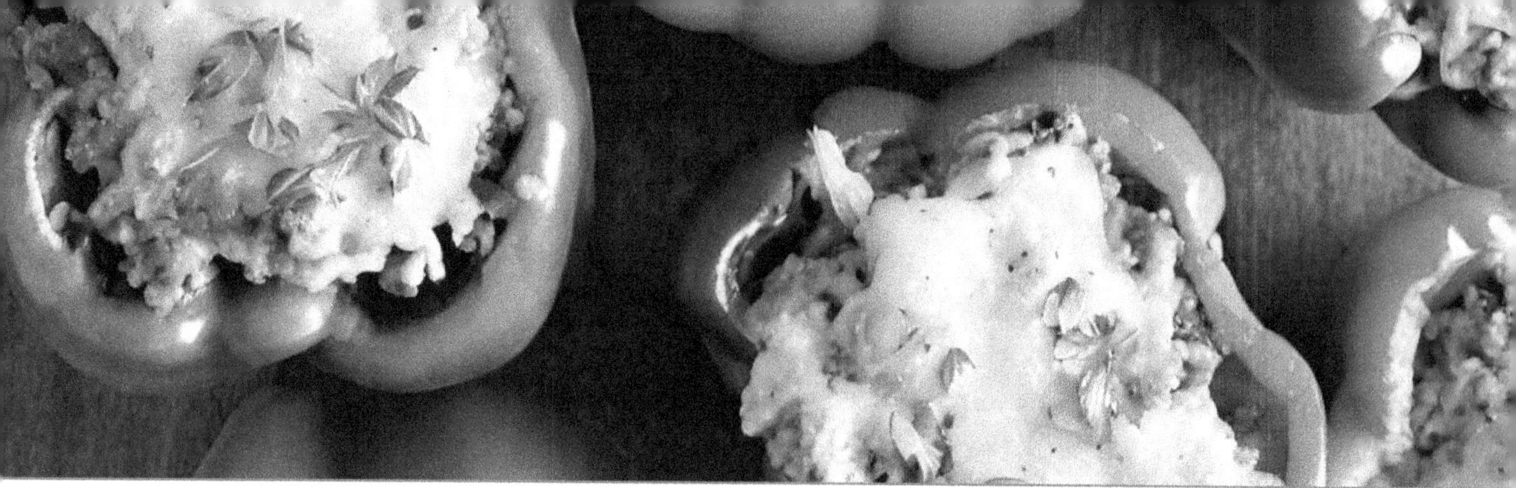

Stuffed Bell Peppers

SERVINGS: 4 PREP TIME: 15 MINUTES COOK TIME: 35-40 MINUTES

INGREDIENTS

- 4 large bell peppers (any color), halved and seeds removed
- 1 lb. (450g) ground turkey or lean ground beef
- 1 cup cauliflower rice
- 1 small onion, finely chopped
- 2 cloves garlic, minced
- 1 cup diced tomatoes (canned or fresh)
- 1/2 cup shredded cheese (such as cheddar or mozzarella)
- 1 teaspoon dried oregano
- 1 teaspoon dried basil
- Salt and pepper to taste
- Olive oil for cooking
- Optional toppings: chopped fresh parsley, grated Parmesan cheese.

INSTRUCTIONS

1. Preheat your oven to 375°F (190°C).
2. Heat olive oil in a skillet over medium heat. Add the chopped onion and minced garlic, and cook until softened, about 3-4 minutes.
3. Add the ground turkey or beef to the skillet and cook until browned, breaking it apart with a spoon.
4. Stir in the cauliflower rice, diced tomatoes, dried oregano, dried basil, salt, and pepper. Cook for another 5 minutes, or until the cauliflower rice is tender and most of the liquid has evaporated.
5. Remove the skillet from the heat and stir in half of the shredded cheese.
6. Place the bell pepper halves in a baking dish, cut side up. Spoon the turkey or beef mixture evenly into each pepper half.
7. Cover the baking dish with aluminum foil and bake in the preheated oven for 25-30 minutes, or until the peppers are tender.

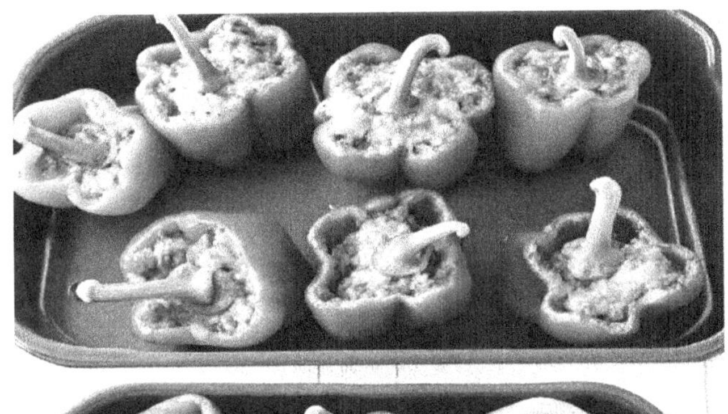

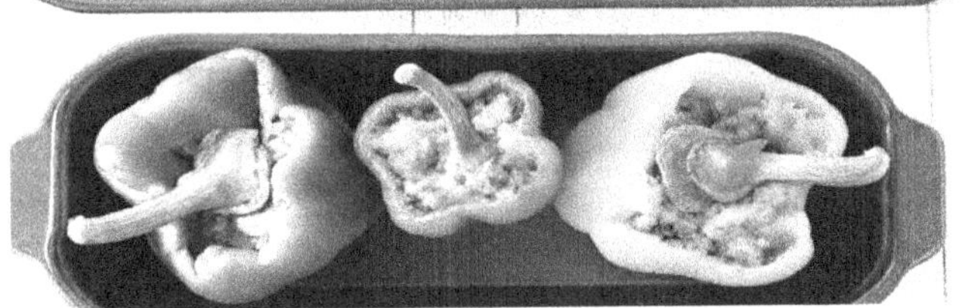

8. Remove the foil and sprinkle the remaining shredded cheese over the stuffed peppers. Return to the oven and bake for an additional 5 minutes, or until the cheese is melted and bubbly.

9. Remove from the oven and let cool slightly before serving.

10. Garnish with chopped fresh parsley and grated Parmesan cheese if desired.

Tips for Variation:

- Add chopped vegetables like mushrooms, zucchini, or spinach to the filling mixture for extra nutrients and flavor.

- Use different types of cheese for variety, such as pepper jack or feta.

- Experiment with different seasonings or sauces to customize the flavor profile, such as taco seasoning for a Tex-Mex twist or Italian seasoning for a Mediterranean flair.

- For a vegetarian option, substitute the ground meat with cooked lentils or quinoa.

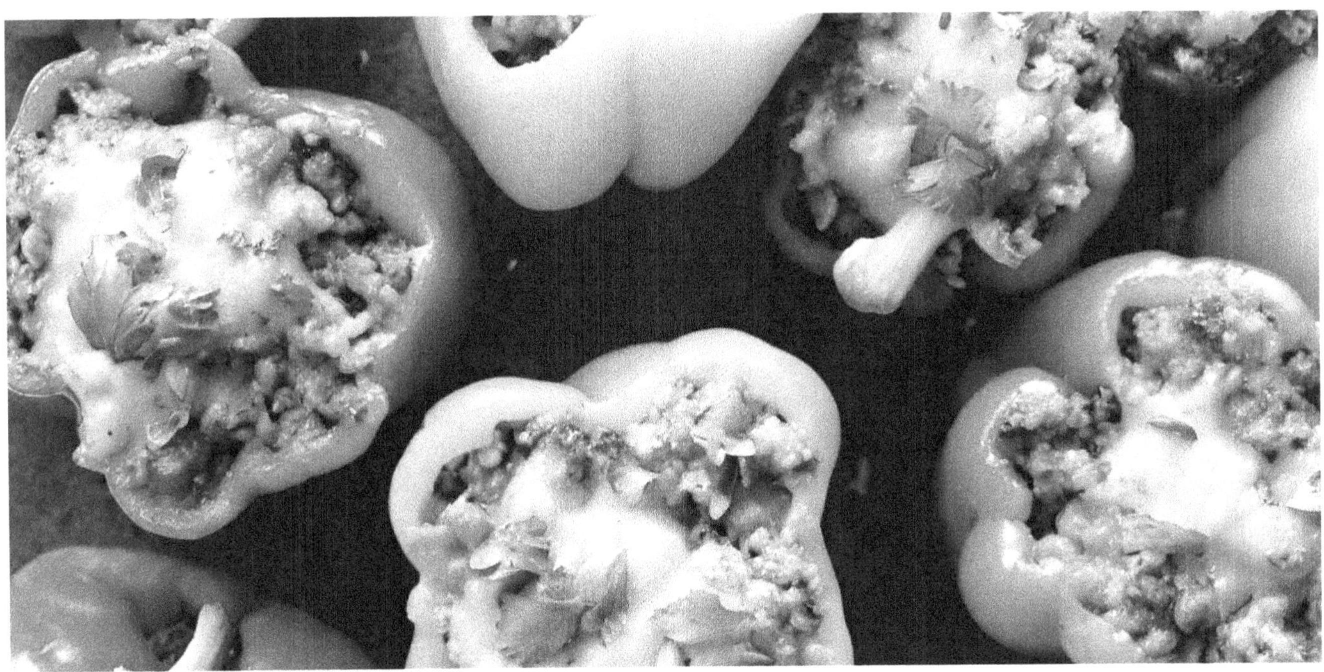

Nutritional Information: *Calories: 290 kcal, Total Fat: 12g, Saturated Fat: 5g, Cholesterol: 80mg, Sodium: 420mg, Total Carbohydrates: 16g, Dietary Fiber: 5g, Sugars: 8g, Protein: 27g*

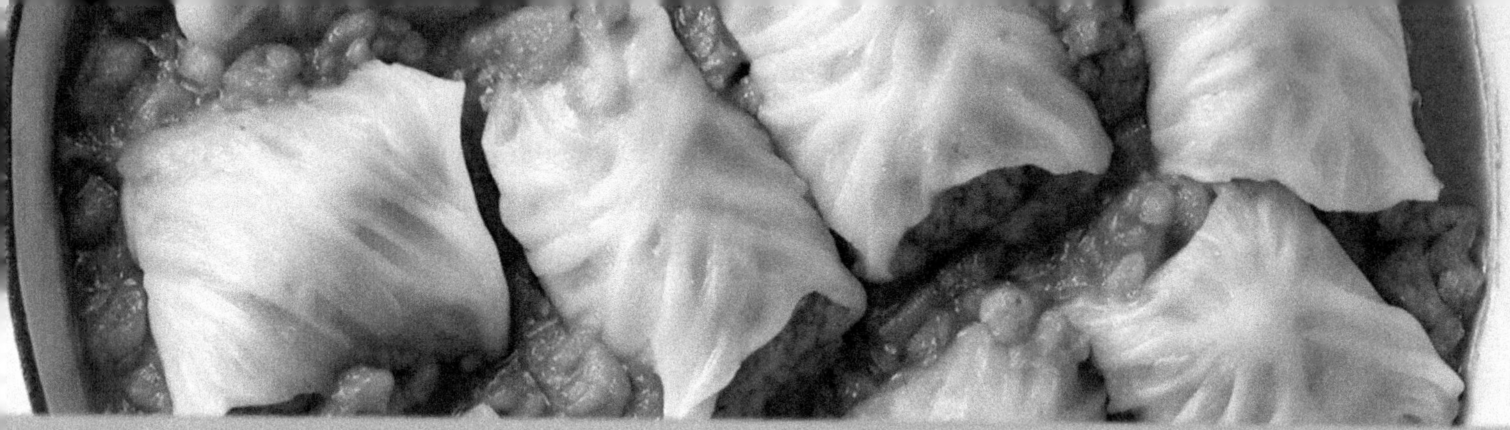

Cabbage Rolls with Ground Beef

SERVINGS: 4-6   PREP TIME: 30 MINUTES   COOK TIME: 1 HOUR

INGREDIENTS

- 1 large head of cabbage
- 1 lb. (450g) lean ground beef
- 1 cup cooked cauliflower rice (or cooked white rice if not following a low-carb diet)
- 1 small onion, finely chopped
- 2 cloves garlic, minced
- 1 (14 oz.) can diced tomatoes
- 1 egg, beaten
- 1 teaspoon dried oregano
- 1 teaspoon dried basil
- Salt and pepper to taste
- 1 cup marinara sauce (homemade or store-bought)
- Fresh parsley for garnish (optional)

INSTRUCTIONS

1. Preheat your oven to 375°F (190°C).
2. Bring a large pot of water to a boil. Carefully remove the core from the cabbage and immerse the whole head of cabbage in the boiling water. Cook for about 5-7 minutes, or until the outer leaves are softened and pliable. Remove the cabbage from the pot and let it cool slightly.
3. In a large skillet, cook the ground beef over medium heat until browned. Add the chopped onion and minced garlic and cook until softened, about 3-4 minutes.
4. Remove the skillet from the heat and stir in the cooked cauliflower rice (or white rice), diced tomatoes (with juices), beaten egg, dried oregano, dried basil, salt, and pepper.
5. Carefully separate the softened cabbage leaves from the head, trimming off any thick ribs if necessary.

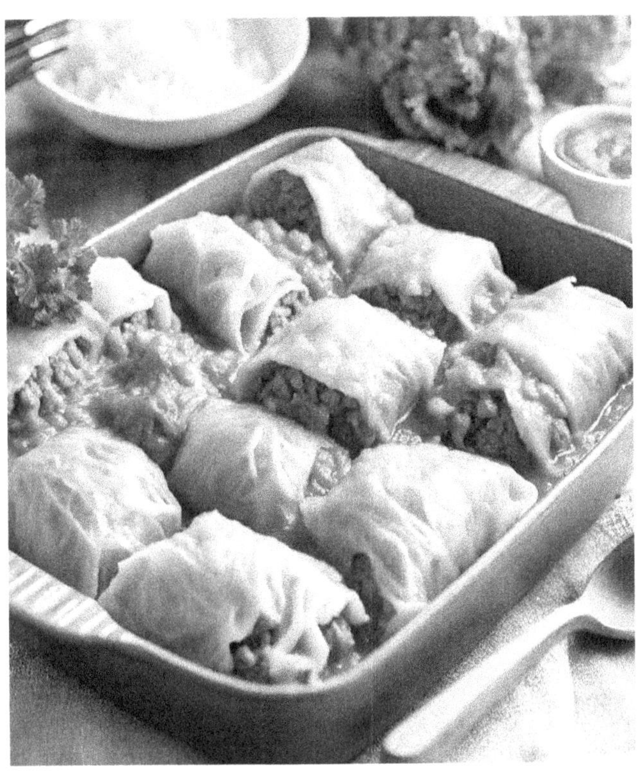

6. Place a spoonful of the ground beef mixture onto each cabbage leaf and roll up tightly, tucking in the sides as you roll. Place the cabbage rolls seam side down in a baking dish.
7. Pour the marinara sauce over the cabbage rolls, covering them evenly.
8. Cover the baking dish with aluminum foil and bake in the preheated oven for 45-50 minutes, or until the cabbage rolls are tender.
9. Remove the foil and bake for an additional 10 minutes to allow the tops to brown slightly.
10. Remove from the oven and let the cabbage rolls cool for a few minutes before serving.
11. Garnish with fresh parsley if desired.

Tips for Variation:

- Use ground turkey or chicken instead of ground beef for a lighter option.
- Add cooked quinoa or lentils to the filling mixture for extra protein and fiber.
- Experiment with different herbs and spices in the filling, such as thyme, rosemary, or paprika.
- Substitute the marinara sauce with a creamy sauce made from Greek yogurt or coconut milk for a different flavor profile.

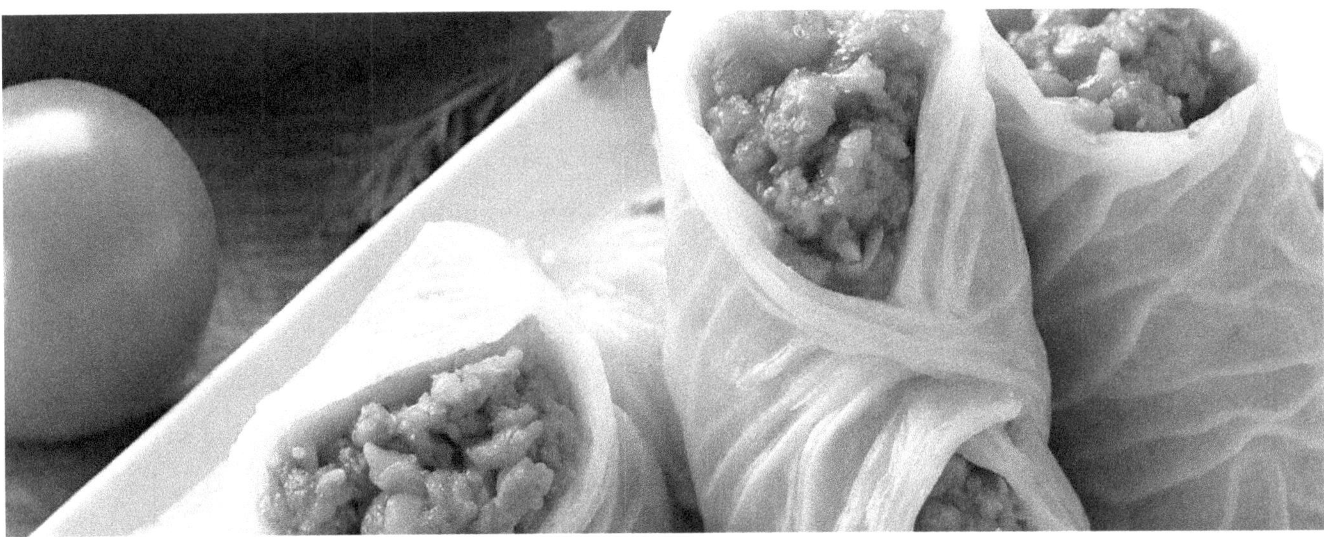

Nutritional Information: *Calories: 250 kcal, Total Fat: 10g, Saturated Fat: 4g, Cholesterol: 80mg, Sodium: 500mg, Total Carbohydrates: 15g, Dietary Fiber: 5g, Sugars: 7g, Protein: 20g*

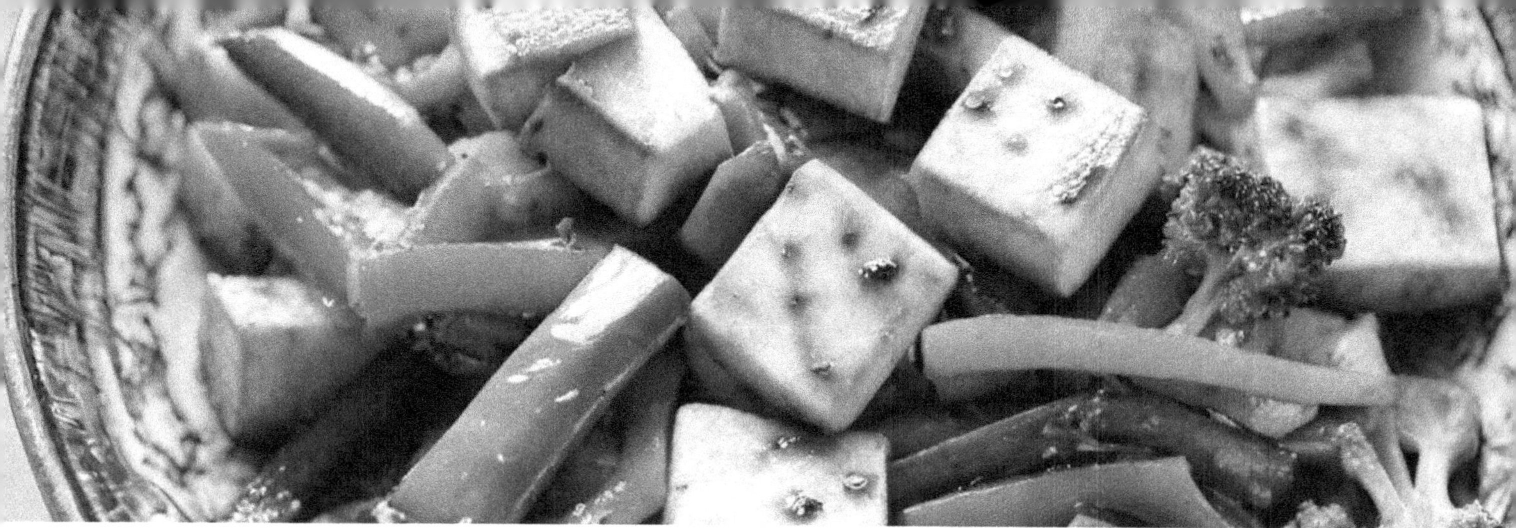

Stir-Fried Tofu with Vegetables

SERVINGS: 4 PREP TIME: 15 MINUTES COOK TIME: 15 MINUTES

INGREDIENTS

- 1 block (14 oz.) firm tofu, drained and pressed
- 2 tablespoons soy sauce (or tamari for gluten-free option)
- 2 tablespoons rice vinegar
- 1 tablespoon sesame oil
- 1 tablespoon cornstarch
- 1 tablespoon olive oil or vegetable oil
- 2 cloves garlic, minced
- 1 tablespoon grated ginger
- 1 bell pepper, thinly sliced
- 1 cup sliced mushrooms
- 1 cup broccoli florets
- 1 carrot, julienned
- Salt and pepper to taste
- Optional garnishes: chopped green onions, sesame seeds

INSTRUCTIONS

1. Cut the pressed tofu into cubes or strips and place them in a bowl. In a separate small bowl, whisk together the soy sauce, rice vinegar, sesame oil, and cornstarch to make the sauce.

2. Heat the olive oil or vegetable oil in a large skillet or wok over medium-high heat. Add the minced garlic and grated ginger, and cook for 1-2 minutes until fragrant.

3. Add the tofu cubes to the skillet in a single layer. Cook for 5-7 minutes, flipping occasionally, until they are golden brown and crispy on all sides. Remove the tofu from the skillet and set aside.

4. In the same skillet, add the sliced bell pepper, mushrooms, broccoli florets, and julienned carrot. Stir-fry for 5-7 minutes, or until the vegetables are tender-crisp.

5. Return the cooked tofu to the skillet with the vegetables. Pour the sauce over the tofu and vegetables, tossing gently to coat everything evenly.

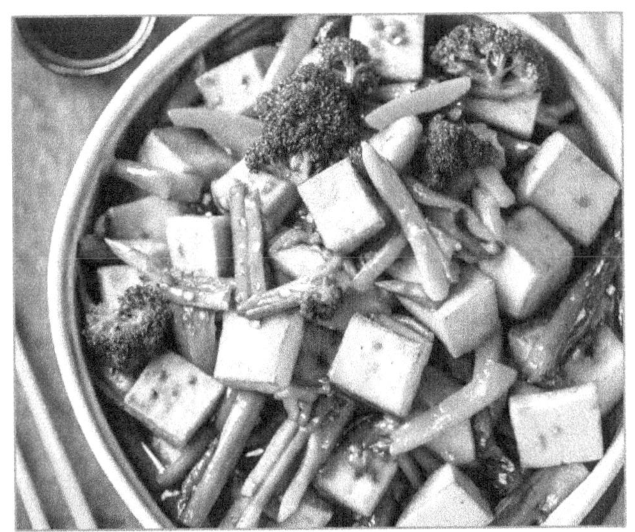

6. Cook for another 2-3 minutes, or until the sauce has thickened slightly.
7. Season with salt and pepper to taste.
8. Serve the stir-fried tofu and vegetables hot, garnished with chopped green onions and sesame seeds if desired.

<u>Tips for Variation:</u>

- Add other vegetables like snow peas, snap peas, baby corn, or water chestnuts for extra crunch and flavor.
- Use different sauces or seasonings for variation, such as teriyaki sauce, hoisin sauce, or chili garlic sauce.
- Substitute tofu with tempeh or seitan for a different plant-based protein option.
- For a heartier meal, serve the stir-fried tofu and vegetables over cooked brown rice or quinoa.

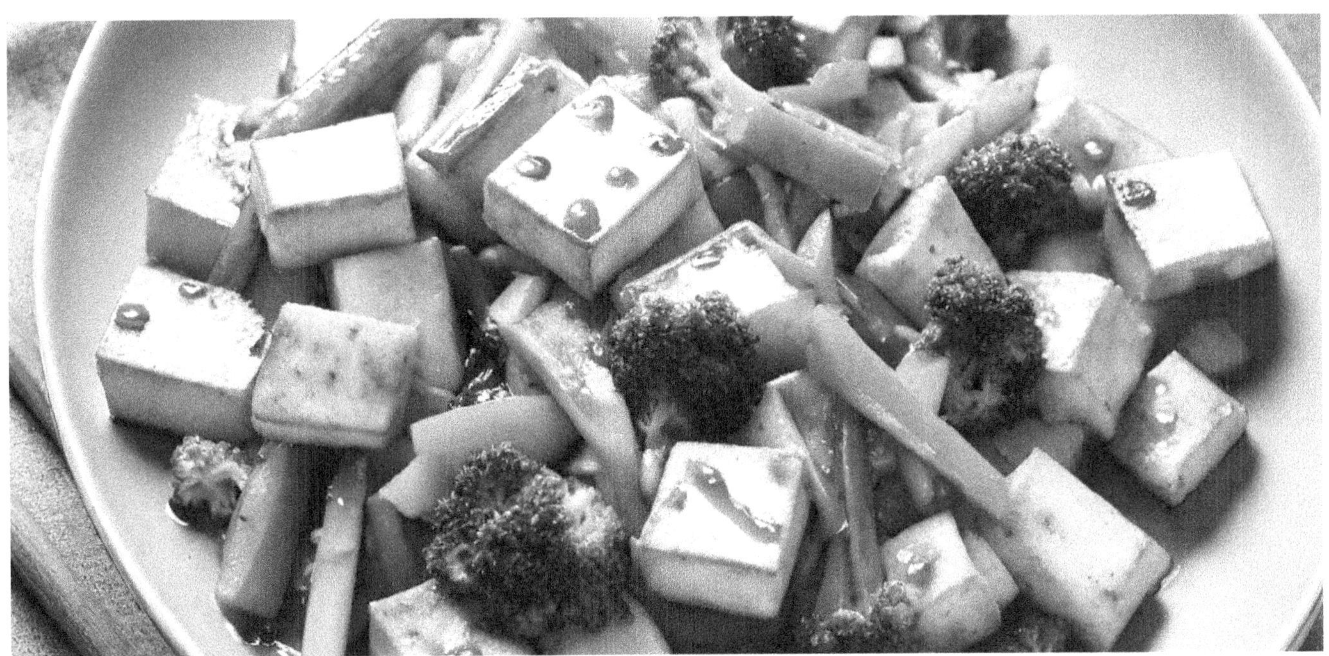

Nutritional Information: *Calories: 220 kcal, Total Fat: 14g, Saturated Fat: 2g, Cholesterol: 0mg, Sodium: 580mg, Total Carbohydrates: 15g, Dietary Fiber: 4g, Sugars: 6g, Protein: 12g*

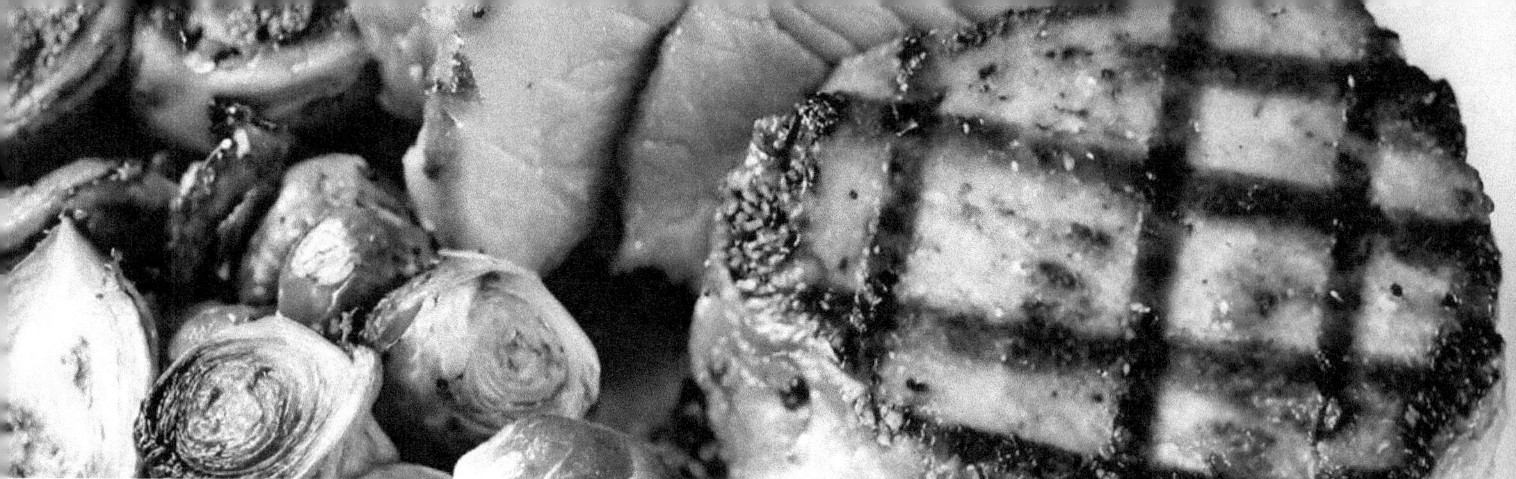

Grilled Pork Chops with Roasted Brussels Sprouts

SERVINGS: 4   PREP TIME: 15 MINUTES   COOK TIME: 30 TO 40 MINUTES

INGREDIENTS

- 4 bone-in pork chops
- Salt and pepper to taste
- 2 tablespoons olive oil
- 1 teaspoon garlic powder
- 1 teaspoon dried thyme
- 1 teaspoon paprika
- 1 lb. (450g) Brussels sprouts, trimmed and halved
- 2 tablespoons balsamic vinegar
- 2 tablespoons honey or low-carb sweetener (such as erythritol or stevia)
- Optional garnish: chopped fresh parsley or thyme

INSTRUCTIONS

1. Preheat your grill to medium-high heat.

2. Season the pork chops with salt, pepper, garlic powder, dried thyme, and paprika. Drizzle with olive oil and rub the seasonings into the meat.

3. Place the seasoned pork chops on the preheated grill and cook for 4-5 minutes per side, or until the internal temperature reaches 145°F (63°C) for medium doneness. Cooking time may vary depending on the thickness of the pork chops.

4. While the pork chops are grilling, preheat your oven to 400°F (200°C).

5. In a large bowl, toss the halved Brussels sprouts with olive oil, salt, and pepper. Spread them out in a single layer on a baking sheet lined with parchment paper.

6. Roast the Brussels sprouts in the preheated oven for 20-25 minutes, or until they are tender and caramelized, stirring halfway through.

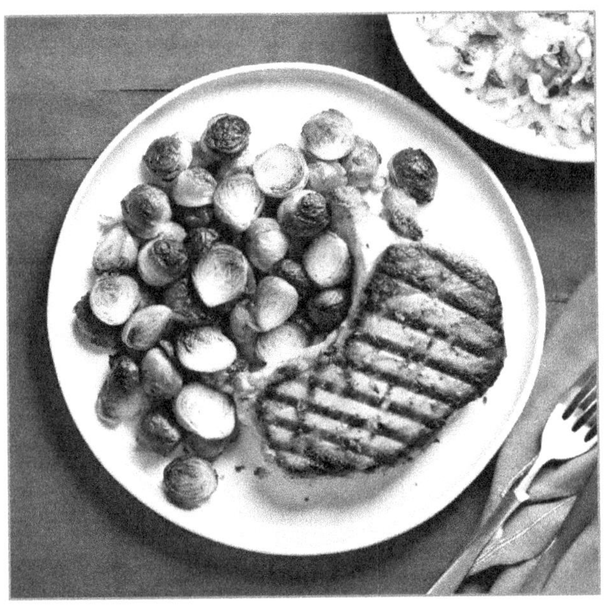

7. In a small saucepan, heat the balsamic vinegar and honey (or low-carb sweetener) over medium heat. Cook for 3-4 minutes, stirring constantly, until the mixture has thickened slightly.

8. Remove the pork chops from the grill and let them rest for a few minutes before serving.

9. Serve the grilled pork chops with the roasted Brussels sprouts, drizzling the balsamic glaze over the top.

10. Garnish with chopped fresh parsley or thyme if desired.

<u>**Tips for Variation:**</u>

- Use boneless pork chops if preferred, adjusting the cooking time as needed.

- Substitute the Brussels sprouts with other roasted vegetables such as carrots, parsnips, or sweet potatoes.

- Make a different glaze for the pork chops using ingredients like maple syrup, mustard, and apple cider vinegar for a sweet and tangy flavor.

- Add a sprinkle of crumbled bacon or toasted nuts over the roasted Brussels sprouts for extra flavor and texture.

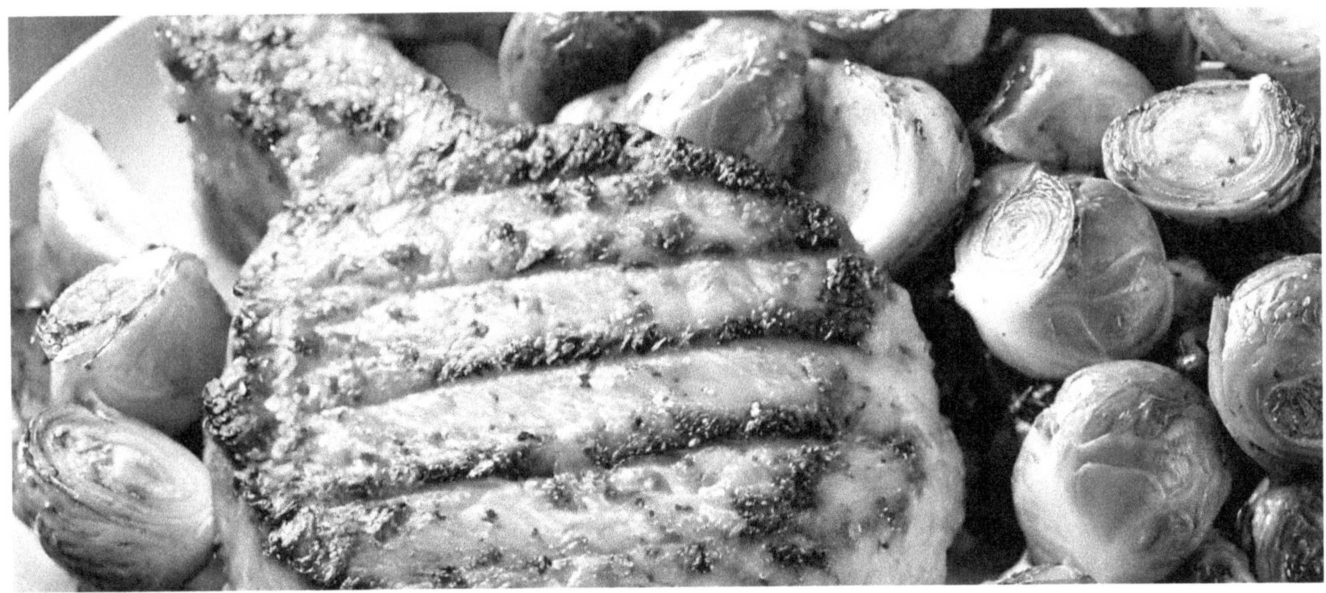

Nutritional Information: *Calories: 380 kcal, Total Fat: 18g, Saturated Fat: 4g, Cholesterol: 90mg, Sodium: 250mg, Total Carbohydrates: 20g, Dietary Fiber: 5g, Sugars: 10g, Protein: 35g*

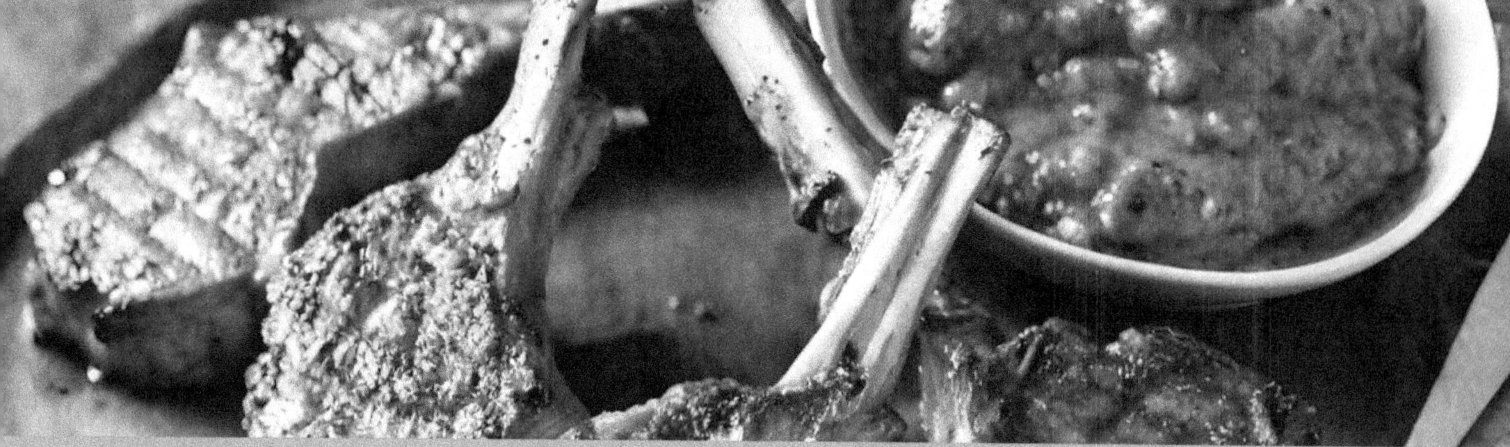

Grilled Lamb Chops with Mint Sauce

SERVINGS: 4　　　　PREP TIME: 10 MINUTES　　　　COOK TIME: 8 TO 10 MINUTES

INGREDIENTS

- 8 lamb chops
- Salt and pepper to taste
- 2 tablespoons olive oil
- 2 cloves garlic, minced
- 1 tablespoon chopped fresh rosemary
- 1 tablespoon chopped fresh thyme
- 1/4 cup chopped fresh mint leaves
- 1/4 cup lemon juice
- 2 tablespoons balsamic vinegar
- 1 tablespoon honey or low-carb sweetener (such as erythritol or stevia)
- Optional garnish: extra chopped fresh mint leaves

INSTRUCTIONS

1. Season the lamb chops with salt and pepper to taste. In a small bowl, mix together the olive oil, minced garlic, chopped rosemary, and chopped thyme. Rub the mixture onto both sides of the lamb chops, coating them evenly. Let them marinate for at least 30 minutes, or refrigerate overnight for more flavor.

2. Preheat your grill to medium-high heat.

3. Place the marinated lamb chops on the preheated grill and cook for 3-4 minutes per side, or until they reach your desired level of doneness. Cooking time may vary depending on the thickness of the lamb chops and your preferred level of doneness.

4. While the lamb chops are grilling, prepare the mint sauce. In a small bowl, combine the chopped mint leaves, lemon juice, balsamic vinegar, and honey (or low-carb sweetener). Stir well to combine.

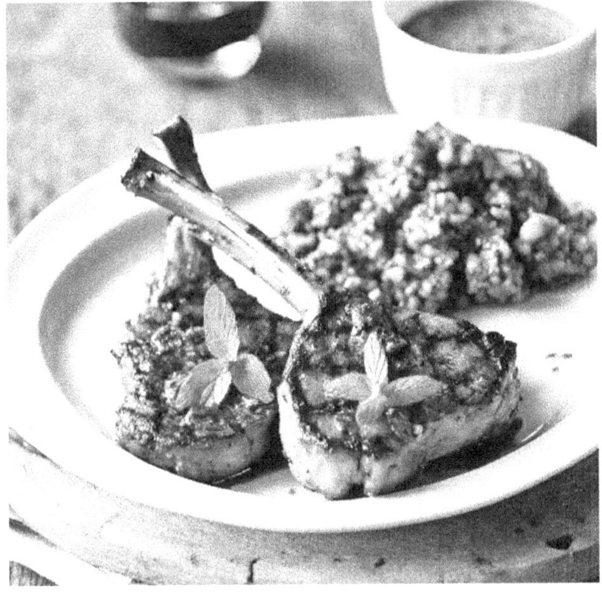

5. Remove the grilled lamb chops from the grill and let them rest for a few minutes before serving.

6. Serve the lamb chops hot, drizzled with the mint sauce. Garnish with extra chopped mint leaves if desired.

Tips for Variation:

- For added flavor, you can add a pinch of ground cumin or coriander to the marinade for the lamb chops.

- If you prefer a smoother mint sauce, you can blend the ingredients together in a food processor or blender until smooth.

- Serve the grilled lamb chops with a side of roasted vegetables or a mixed green salad for a complete meal.

- Substitute the mint sauce with a different sauce or condiment, such as tzatziki or chimichurri, for a different flavor profile.

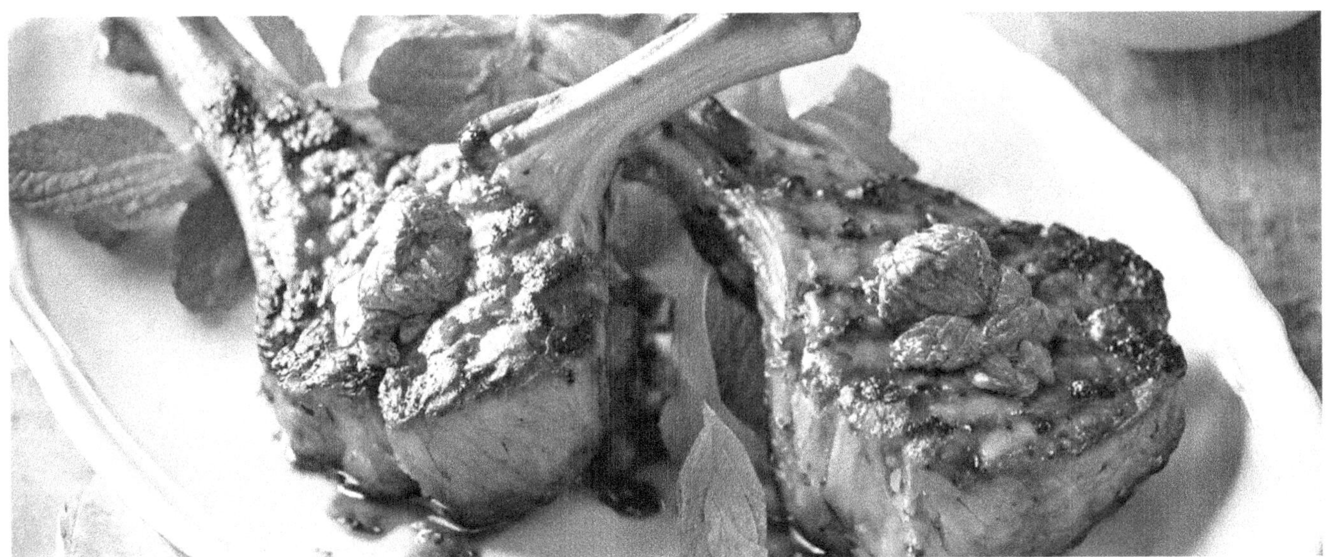

Nutritional Information: *Calories: 380 kcal, Total Fat: 22g, Saturated Fat: 8g, Cholesterol: 120mg, Sodium: 75mg, Total Carbohydrates: 5g, Dietary Fiber: 1g, Sugars: 3g, Protein: 38g*

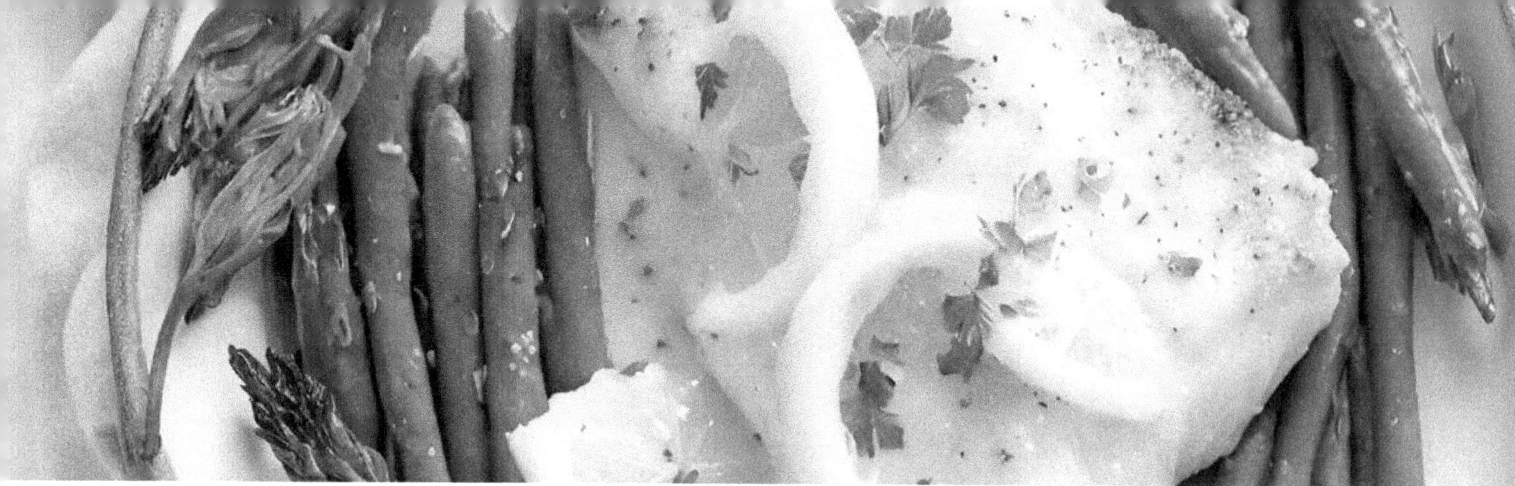

Baked Cod with Lemon Butter Sauce

SERVINGS: 4   PREP TIME: 10 MINUTES   COOK TIME: 12 TO 15 MINUTES

INGREDIENTS

- 4 cod fillets (about 6 ounces each)
- Salt and pepper to taste
- 2 tablespoons olive oil
- 2 cloves garlic, minced
- 2 tablespoons fresh lemon juice
- 1/4 cup chicken broth
- 2 tablespoons unsalted butter
- 1 tablespoon chopped fresh parsley
- Lemon slices for garnish (optional)

INSTRUCTIONS

1. Preheat your oven to 400°F (200°C). Grease a baking dish with olive oil or non-stick spray.
2. Pat the cod fillets dry with paper towels and season both sides with salt and pepper. Place the fillets in the prepared baking dish.
3. In a small saucepan, heat the olive oil over medium heat. Add the minced garlic and cook for 1-2 minutes until fragrant.
4. Stir in the fresh lemon juice and chicken broth. Bring the mixture to a simmer and cook for another 2-3 minutes.
5. Remove the saucepan from the heat and stir in the unsalted butter until melted and combined. Season with salt and pepper to taste.
6. Pour the lemon butter sauce over the cod fillets in the baking dish.
7. Bake the cod in the preheated oven for 12-15 minutes, or until the fish flakes easily with a fork and is cooked through.

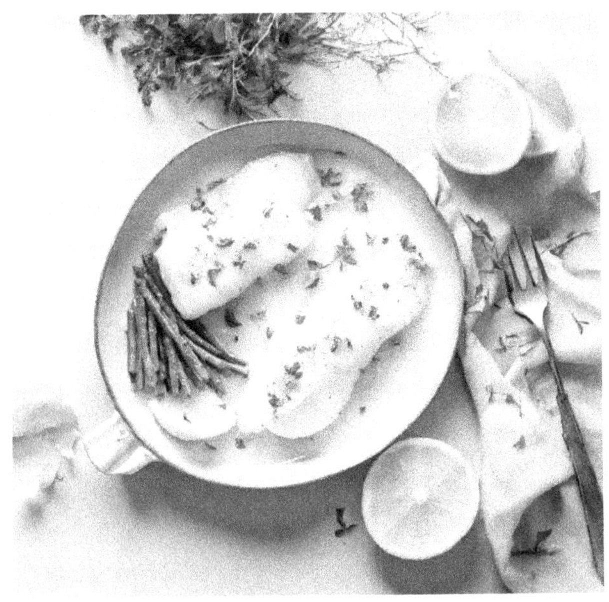

8. Remove the baked cod from the oven and sprinkle with chopped fresh parsley.

9. Serve hot, garnished with lemon slices if desired.

Tips for Variation:

- Add additional herbs or spices to the lemon butter sauce, such as dill, tarragon, or crushed red pepper flakes, for extra flavor.

- Substitute the cod fillets with other types of white fish, such as haddock, halibut, or tilapia.

- For a low-carb option, use vegetable broth instead of chicken broth in the lemon butter sauce.

- Serve the baked cod with a side of roasted vegetables, steamed asparagus, or a mixed green salad for a complete meal.

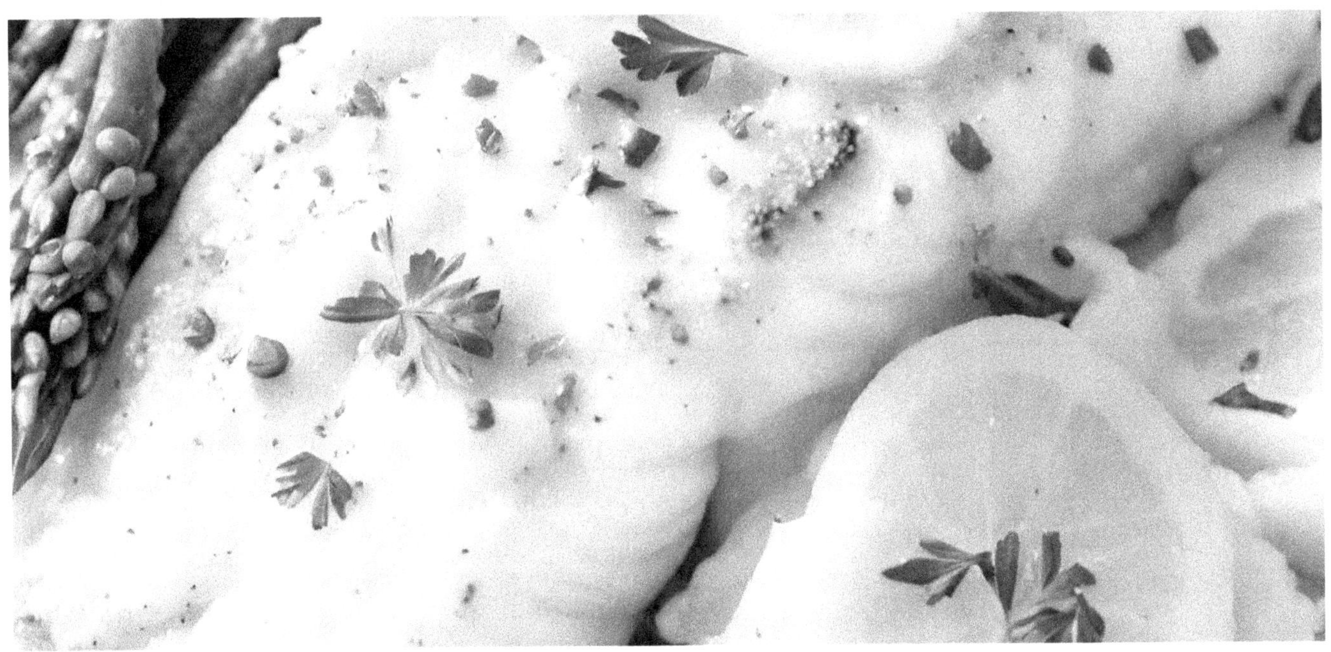

Nutritional Information: *Calories: 260 kcal, Total Fat: 14g, Saturated Fat: 5g, Cholesterol: 85mg, Sodium: 280mg, Total Carbohydrates: 2g, Dietary Fiber: 0g, Sugars: 0g, Protein: 30g*

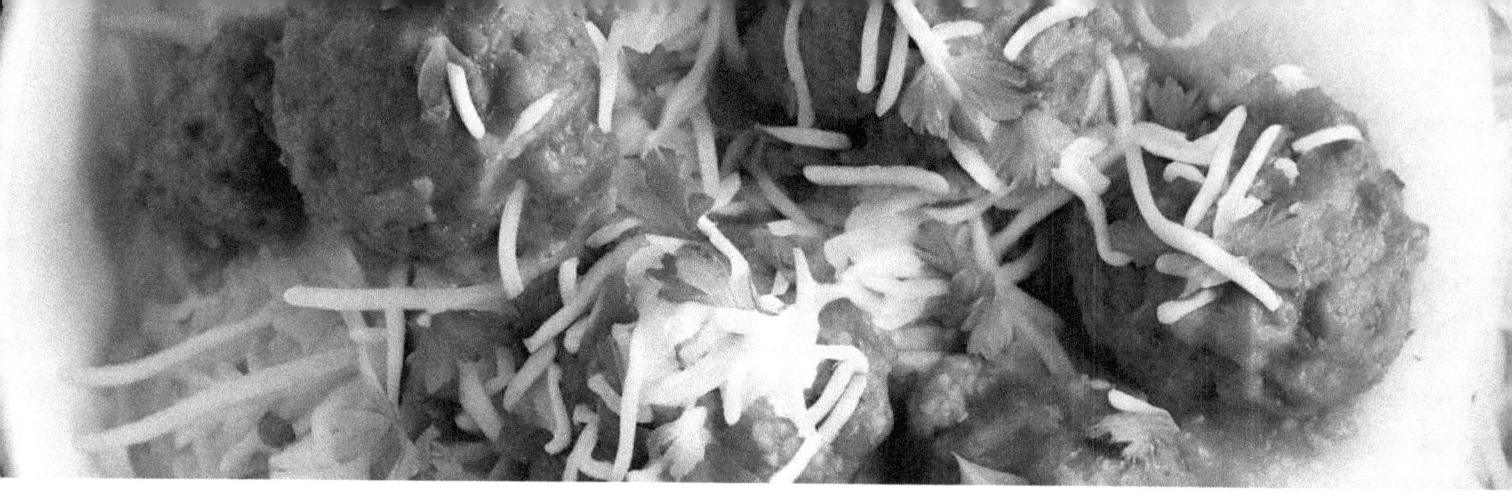

Spaghetti Squash with Meatballs

SERVINGS: 4   PREP TIME: 10 MINUTES   COOK TIME: 40 MINUTES TO 1 HR.

INGREDIENTS

INSTRUCTIONS

For the Spaghetti Squash:

- 1 large spaghetti squash
- Salt and pepper to taste
- Olive oil

For the Meatballs:

- 1 lb. (450g) ground beef
- 1/4 cup almond flour (or breadcrumbs if not following a low-carb diet)
- 1/4 cup grated Parmesan cheese
- 1 egg
- 2 cloves garlic, minced
- 1 teaspoon dried oregano
- 1 teaspoon dried basil
- Salt and pepper to taste)

For the Marinara Sauce:

- 1 (14 oz.) can crushed tomatoes
- 2 cloves garlic, minced

1. Preheat your oven to 400°F (200°C).

2. Cut the spaghetti squash in half lengthwise and scoop out the seeds. Brush the cut sides with olive oil and season with salt and pepper. Place the squash halves cut side down on a baking sheet lined with parchment paper. Bake in the preheated oven for 40-45 minutes, or until the squash is tender and easily pierced with a fork.

3. While the spaghetti squash is baking, prepare the meatballs. In a large mixing bowl, combine the ground beef, almond flour, grated Parmesan cheese, egg, minced garlic, dried oregano, dried basil, salt, and pepper. Mix until well combined. Shape the mixture into meatballs, about 1-2 inches in diameter.

4. Heat a drizzle of olive oil in a large skillet over medium heat. Add the meatballs to the skillet and cook for 8-10 minutes, turning occasionally, until browned on all sides and cooked through.

- 1 teaspoon dried oregano
- 1 teaspoon dried basil
- Salt and pepper to taste
- Fresh basil leaves for garnish (optional)

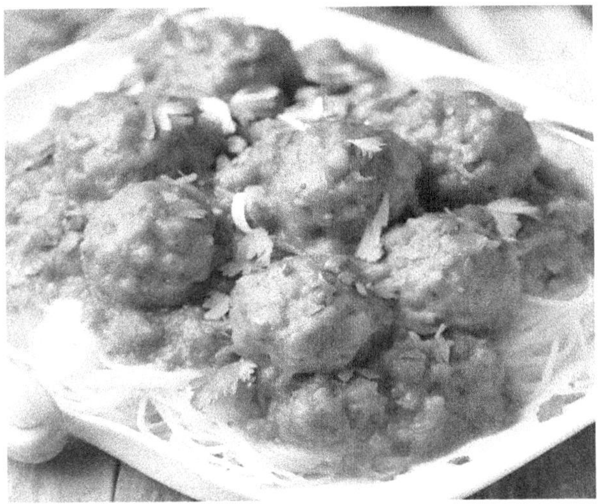

5. In a separate saucepan, prepare the marinara sauce. Heat a little olive oil over medium heat and add the minced garlic. Cook for 1-2 minutes until fragrant. Stir in the crushed tomatoes, dried oregano, dried basil, salt, and pepper. Simmer for 10-15 minutes, stirring occasionally, until the sauce has thickened slightly.
6. Once the spaghetti squash is done baking, use a fork to scrape the flesh into strands. Divide the spaghetti squash strands among serving plates.
7. Top the spaghetti squash with the cooked meatballs and marinara sauce.
8. Garnish with fresh basil leaves if desired and serve hot.

Tips for Variation:

- Use ground turkey or chicken instead of ground beef for a lighter option.
- Add chopped fresh parsley or basil to the meatball mixture for extra flavor.
- Experiment with different seasonings or herbs in the marinara sauce, such as red pepper flakes for a spicy kick or fresh thyme for a more herbal flavor.
- Substitute the spaghetti squash with spiralized zucchini noodles or shirataki noodles for a low-carb alternative.

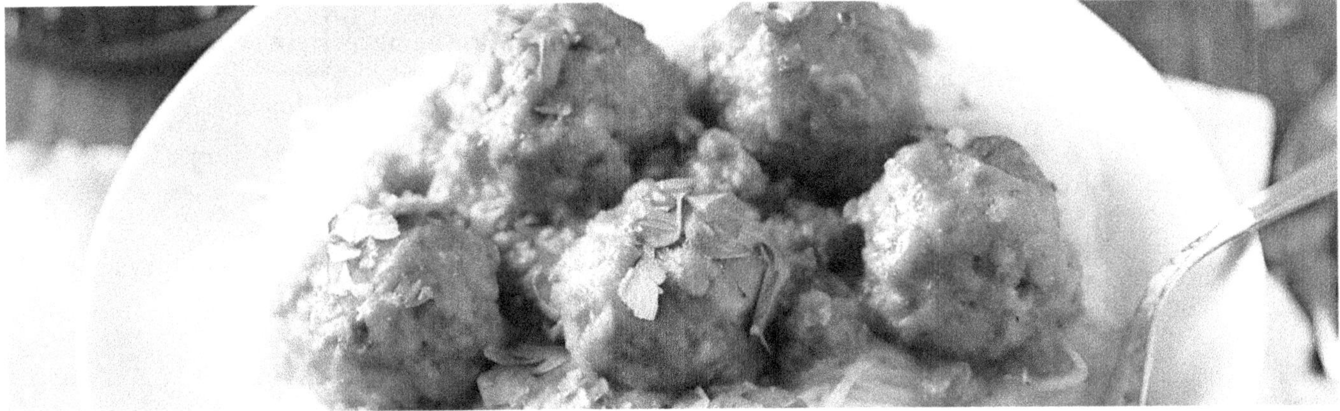

Nutritional Information (per serving, including meatballs and marinara sauce): *Calories: 380 kcal, Total Fat: 20g, Saturated Fat: 7g, Cholesterol: 120mg, Sodium: 700mg, Total Carbohydrates: 18g, Dietary Fiber: 5g, Sugars: 8g, Protein: 30g*

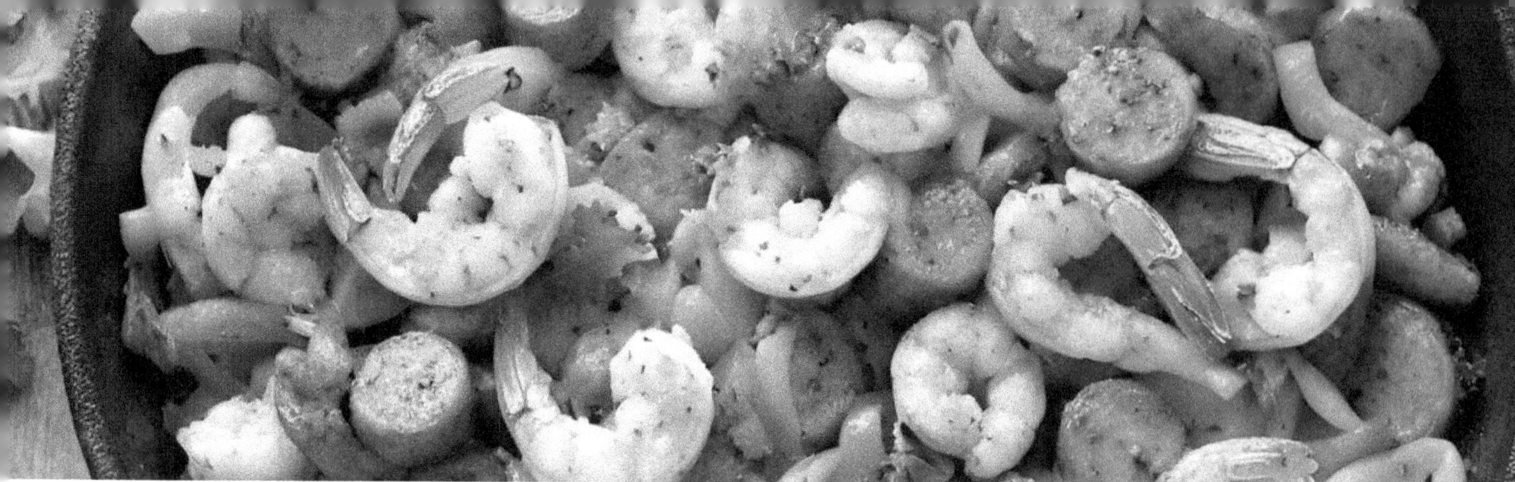

Cajun Shrimp and Sausage Skillet

SERVINGS: 4   PREP TIME: 10 MINUTES   COOK TIME: 15 MINUTES

INGREDIENTS

- 1 lb. (450g) large shrimp, peeled and deveined
- 12 oz. (340g) smoked sausage, sliced into rounds
- 1 bell pepper, sliced
- 1 onion, sliced
- 2 cloves garlic, minced
- 1 tablespoon Cajun seasoning
- 1 teaspoon paprika
- 1/2 teaspoon dried thyme
- Salt and pepper to taste
- 2 tablespoons olive oil
- Fresh parsley for garnish (optional)
- Cooked rice or cauliflower rice for serving (optional)

INSTRUCTIONS

1. In a small bowl, combine the Cajun seasoning, paprika, dried thyme, salt, and pepper.
2. Heat the olive oil in a large skillet over medium-high heat. Add the sliced sausage to the skillet and cook for 3-4 minutes, stirring occasionally, until browned.
3. Add the sliced bell pepper and onion to the skillet and cook for another 3-4 minutes, until softened.
4. Stir in the minced garlic and cook for 1 minute until fragrant.
5. Add the Cajun seasoning mixture to the skillet and stir to coat the sausage, bell pepper, and onion evenly.
6. Push the sausage and vegetables to one side of the skillet and add the shrimp to the other side. Cook the shrimp for 2-3 minutes per side, or until they are pink and opaque.
7. Once the shrimp are cooked through, stir everything together in the skillet to combine.
8. Remove the skillet from the heat and garnish with chopped fresh parsley if desired.

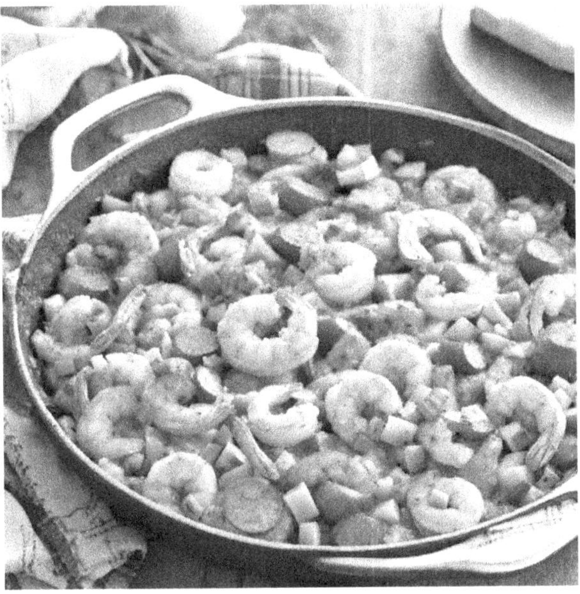

9. Serve the Cajun shrimp and sausage skillet hot, either on its own or over cooked rice or cauliflower rice.

Tips for Variation:

- Add diced tomatoes or tomato sauce to the skillet for extra moisture and flavor.
- Include other vegetables such as zucchini, cherry tomatoes, or mushrooms for added nutrients and variety.
- Use different types of sausage such as andouille sausage or chorizo for a spicier flavor profile.
- Adjust the level of Cajun seasoning according to your preference for heat and spice.
- Serve the Cajun shrimp and sausage skillet with crusty bread or cornbread for a hearty meal.

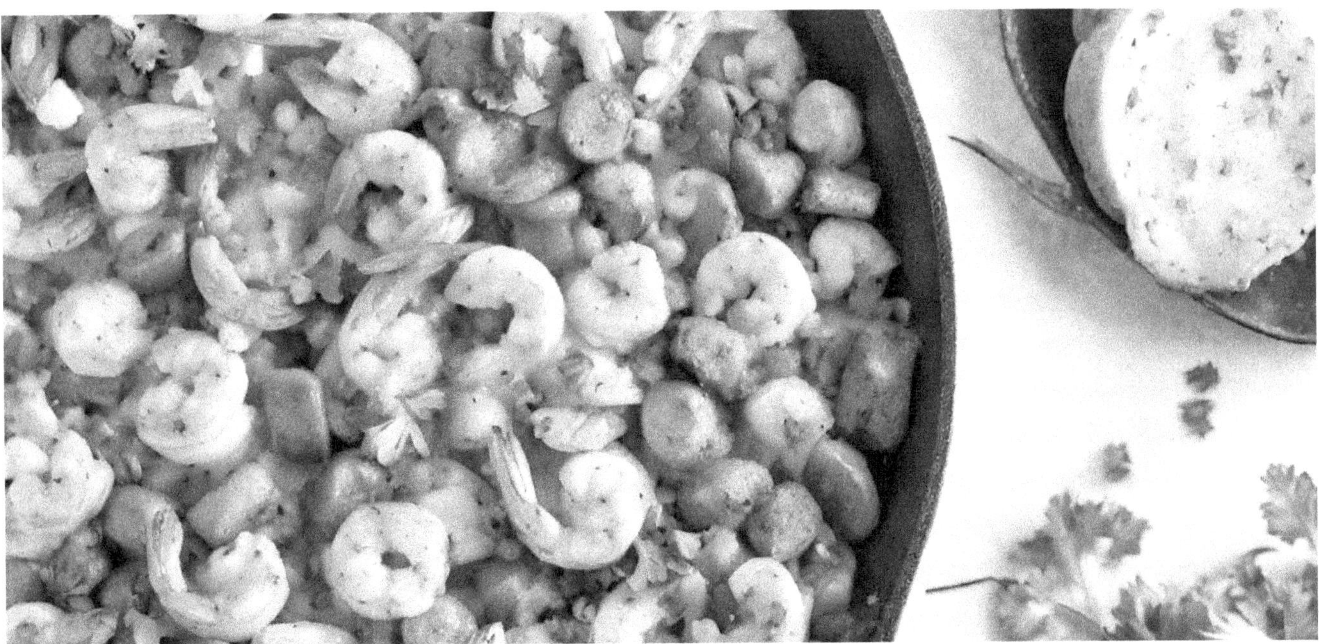

Nutritional Information: *Calories: 380 kcal, Total Fat: 24g, Saturated Fat: 7g, Cholesterol: 260mg, Sodium: 1000mg, Total Carbohydrates: 10g, Dietary Fiber: 2g, Sugars: 4g, Protein: 30g*

Notes:

Your
Observation:

Progress
Report:

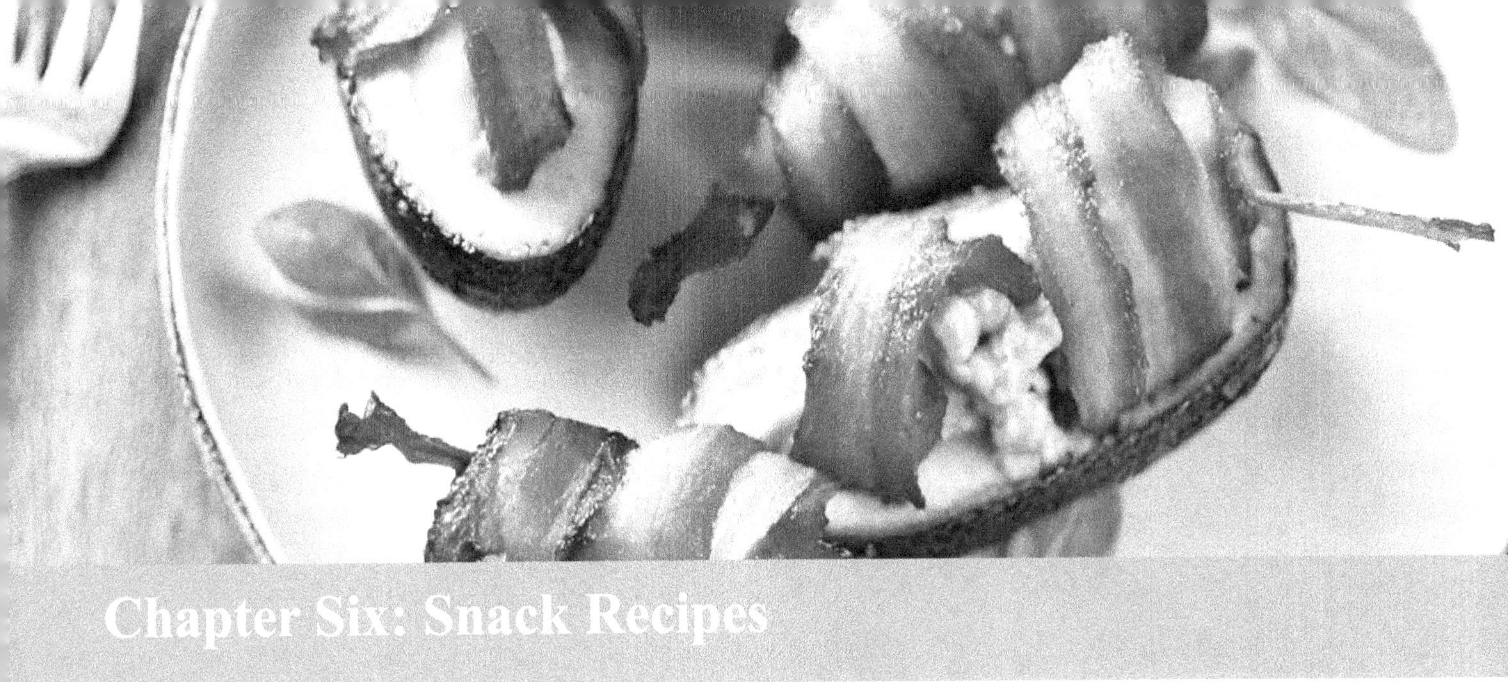

Phase 1: Induction Recipes

Bacon-Wrapped Avocado

SERVINGS: 4 PREP TIME: 10 MINUTES COOK TIME: 15 TO 20 MINUTES

- 2 ripe avocados
- 4 slices of bacon (choose sugar-free bacon if available)
- Salt and black pepper to taste
- Toothpicks (for securing bacon)

1. Preheat your oven to 375°F (190°C).

2. Cut the ripe avocados in half and remove the pit. Carefully peel off the skin and cut each avocado half into two or three wedges, depending on the size.

3. Wrap each avocado wedge with a slice of bacon, securing it with a toothpick. You can either wrap the entire wedge or just a portion, depending on your preference.

4. Sprinkle a pinch of salt and black pepper over the bacon-wrapped avocado for added flavor.

5. Place the bacon-wrapped avocado on a baking sheet lined with parchment paper to prevent sticking.

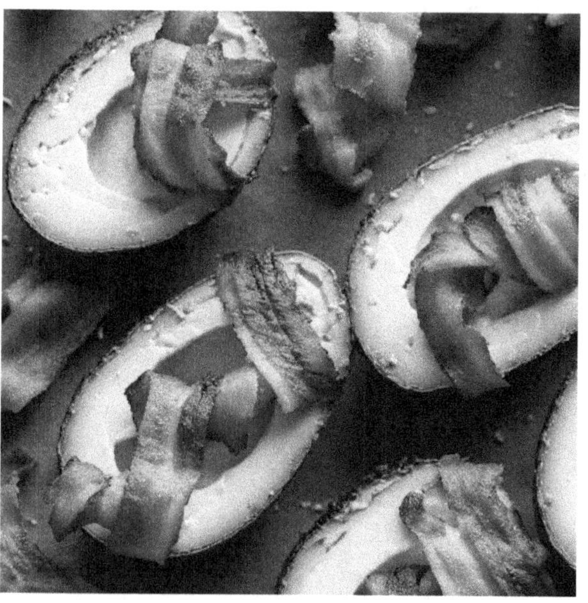

6. Bake in the preheated oven for about 15-20 minutes or until the bacon becomes crispy and the avocado is heated through.

7. Remove the toothpicks before serving. You can enjoy these bacon-wrapped avocado bites hot or at room temperature

Tips for Variation:

- Add a sprinkle of chili powder or smoked paprika for a spicy kick.

- For extra flavor, brush the bacon-wrapped avocado with a bit of olive oil or melted butter before baking.

- Serve with a side of low-carb ranch dressing or your favorite dipping sauce.

- Experiment with different types of bacon, such as turkey bacon or beef bacon, for variety. Just be sure to check the carb content and choose sugar-free options when following the Atkins Diet.

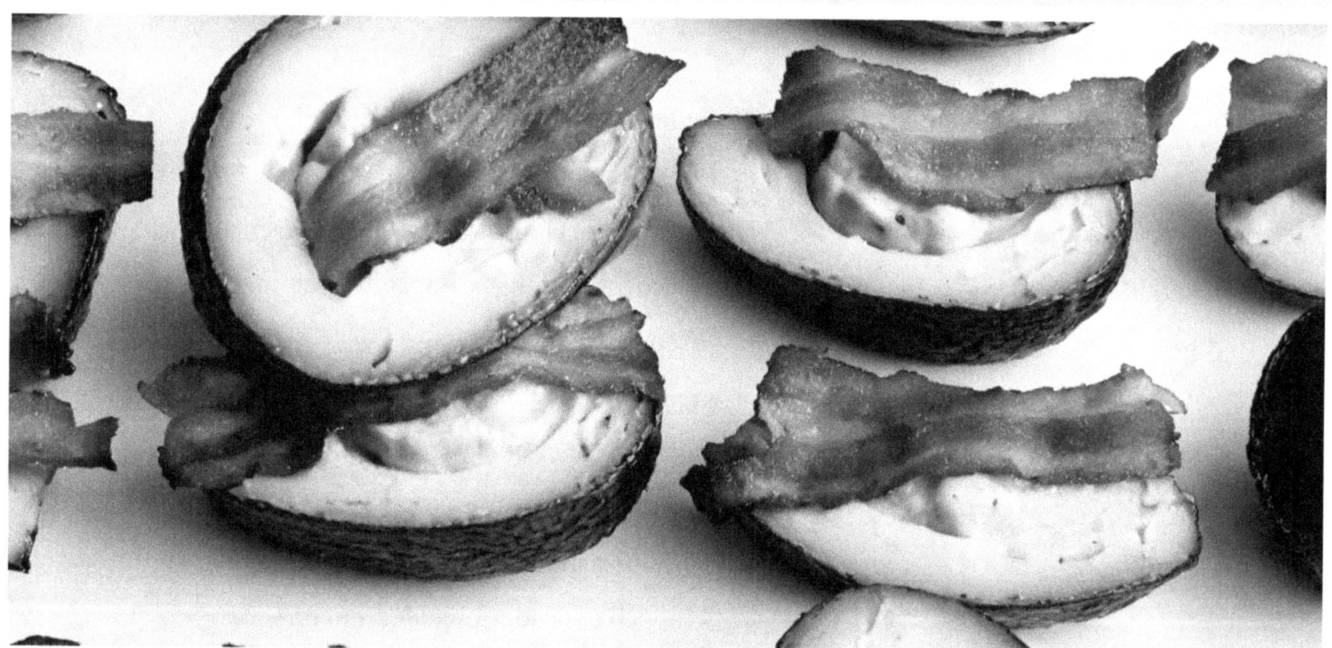

Nutritional Information: *Calories: 185 calories, Total Fat: 15g, Saturated Fat: 3g, Cholesterol: 15mg, Sodium: 250mg, Total Carbohydrates: 7g, Dietary Fiber: 5g, Sugars: 0.5g, Protein: 6g*

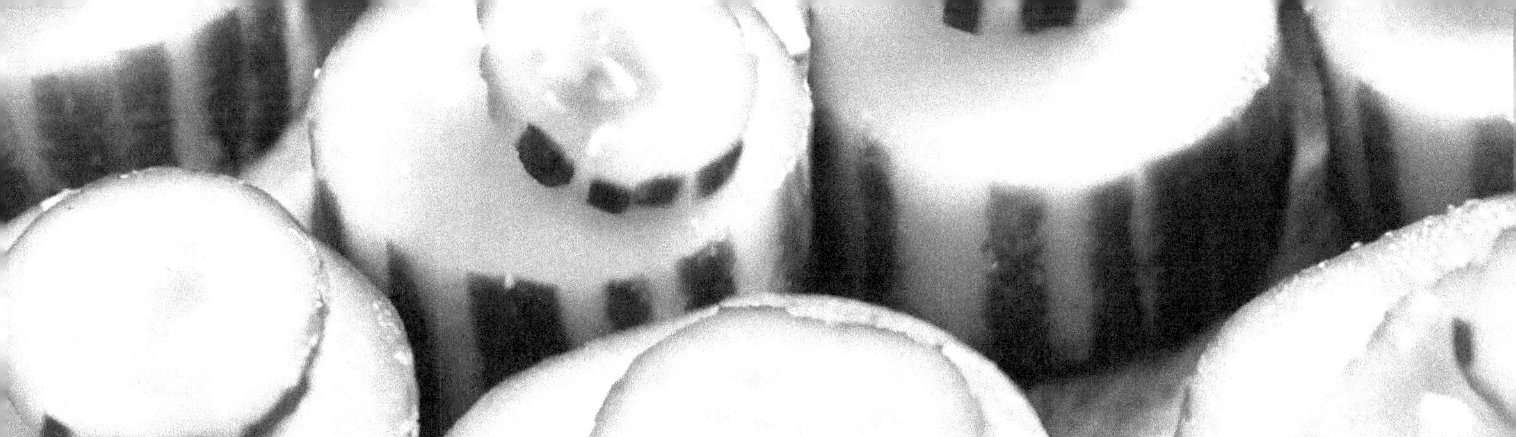

Cucumber Bites

- 2 medium-sized cucumbers
- 4 oz. (113g) smoked salmon
- 4 oz. (113g) cream cheese
- 1/4 teaspoon black pepper (optional)
- Fresh dill or chives for garnish (optional)

Tips for Variation:

- Add a squeeze of fresh lemon juice or a bit of lemon zest to brighten up the flavors.
- Include a thin slice of red onion for a subtle kick.
- Use flavored cream cheese, such as chive and onion or garlic and herb, to add extra flavor.
- Experiment with different smoked fish options like trout or mackerel if you prefer alternatives to salmon.

1. Wash and peel the cucumbers. Slice them into rounds, each about 1/4-inch thick.
2. Cut the smoked salmon into small pieces that will fit nicely on top of the cucumber rounds.
3. Soften the cream cheese by leaving it out at room temperature for a little while or using a microwave on low power for a few seconds.
4. Take a cucumber round and place a small amount of softened cream cheese on top (about 1/2 teaspoon). Add a piece of smoked salmon on top of the cream cheese. If desired, sprinkle a pinch of black pepper for extra flavor.
5. Garnish each cucumber bite with a small sprig of fresh dill or some chopped chives for added freshness and visual appeal.
6. Arrange the cucumber bites on a serving platter and serve immediately.

Nutritional Information: *Calories: 90 calories, Total Fat: 7g, Saturated Fat: 2g, Cholesterol: 190mg, Sodium: 190mg, Total Carbohydrates: 0.5g, Dietary Fiber: 0g, Sugars: 0g, Protein: 6g*

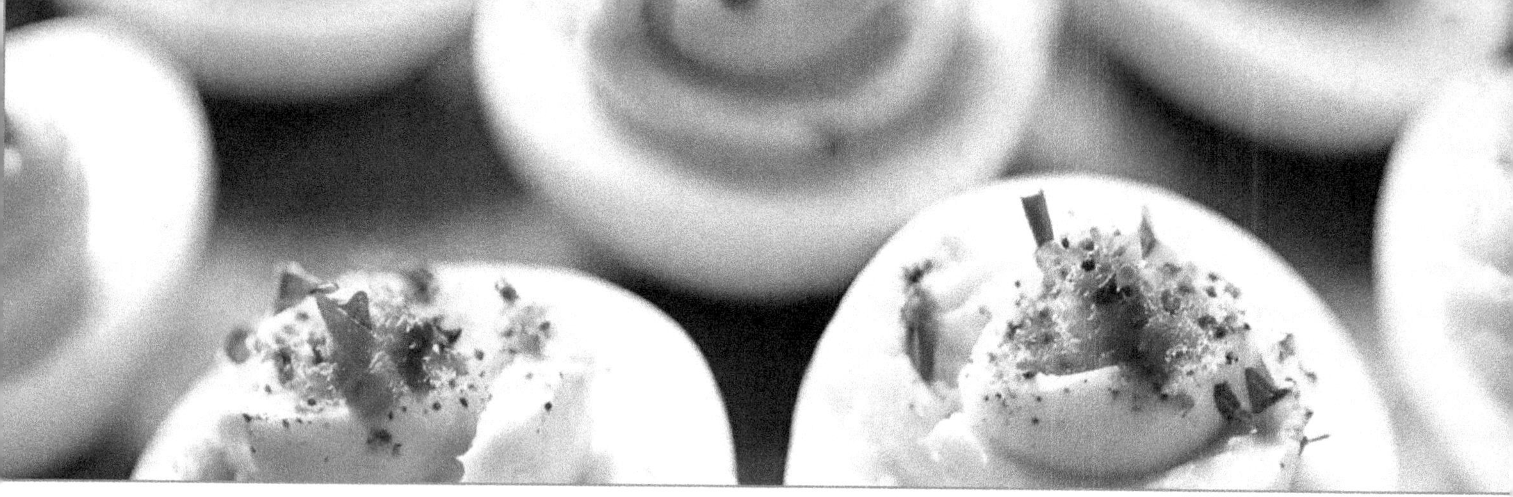

Deviled Eggs

SERVINGS: 6   PREP TIME: 20 MINUTES   COOK TIME: 12 MINUTES

INGREDIENTS

6 large eggs

2 tablespoons mayonnaise (sugar-free)

1 teaspoon Dijon mustard

1/4 teaspoon salt

1/4 teaspoon black pepper

Paprika (for garnish, optional)

Chopped fresh chives or parsley (for garnish, optional)

INSTRUCTIONS

1. Place the eggs in a saucepan and cover them with water. Bring the water to a boil over high heat. Once boiling, reduce the heat to low, cover, and simmer for 10-12 minutes.

2. After boiling, remove the eggs from the heat and place them in a bowl of ice water for about 5 minutes to cool and stop the cooking process.

3. Gently tap each egg on a hard surface to crack the shell, then peel the eggs carefully. Rinse them to remove any remaining shell fragments.

4. Cut each egg in half lengthwise. Carefully remove the yolks and place them in a separate bowl. Arrange the egg white halves on a serving platter.

5. Mash the egg yolks with a fork, and then add mayonnaise, Dijon mustard, salt, and black pepper. Mix until the filling is smooth and well combined.

6. Spoon or pipe the yolk mixture back into the egg white halves. You can use a pastry bag with a decorative tip for a more visually appealing presentation.

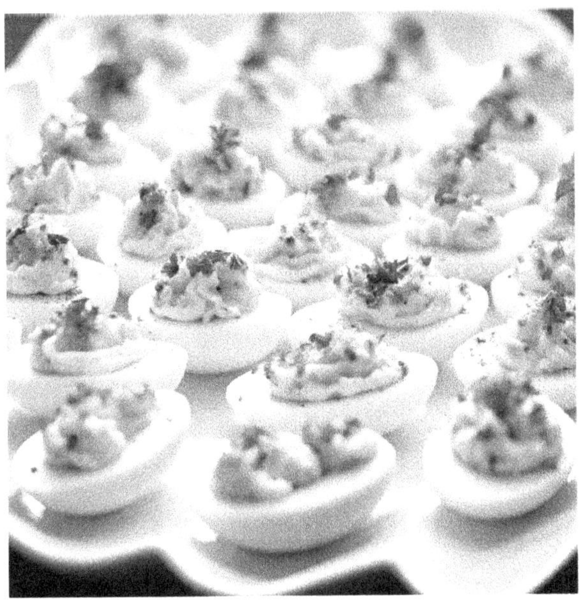

7. If desired, sprinkle a pinch of paprika over each deviled egg for color and flavor. You can also garnish with chopped fresh chives or parsley.

8. Refrigerate the deviled eggs for at least 30 minutes before serving to allow the flavors to meld. Serve chilled.

Tips for Variation:

- Add a dash of hot sauce or cayenne pepper for a spicy kick.
- Mix in finely chopped pickles, olives, or capers for added texture and flavor.
- Garnish with bacon bits for a smoky twist.
- Experiment with different types of mustard, such as whole-grain or spicy brown mustard, for unique flavor profiles.

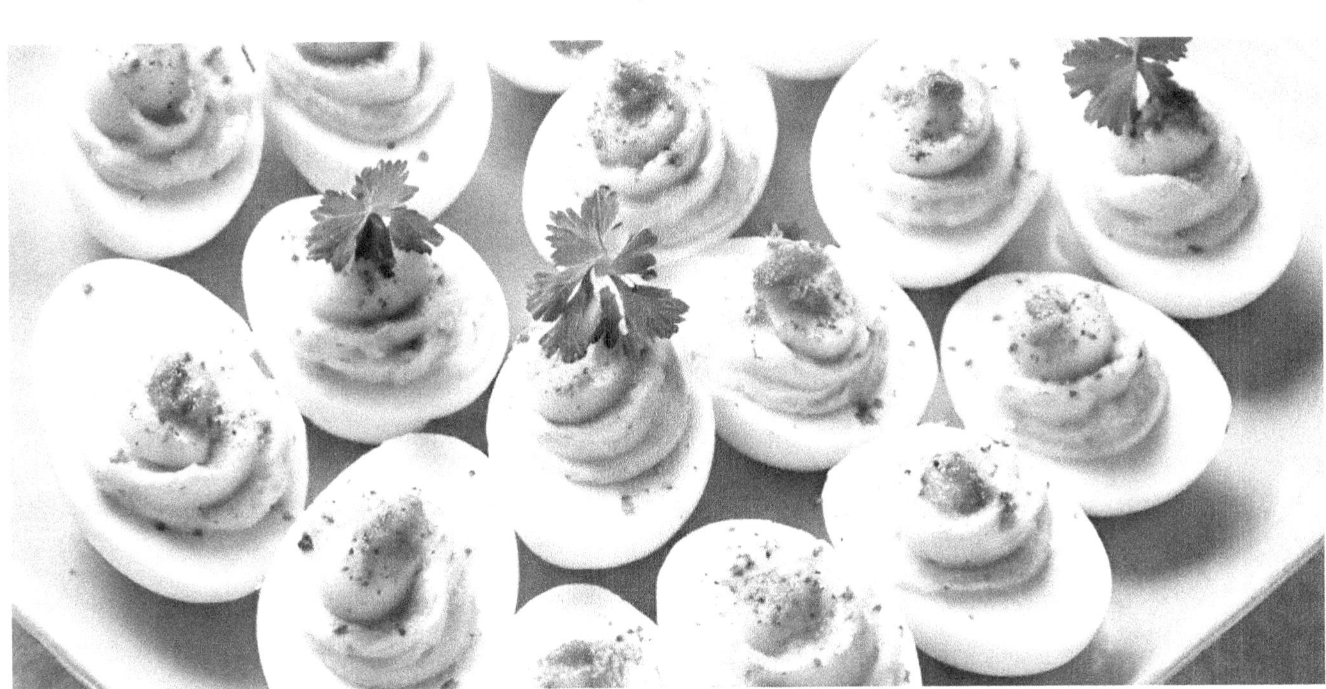

Nutritional Information: *Calories: 90 calories, Total Fat: 7g, Saturated Fat: 2g, Cholesterol: 190mg, Sodium: 190mg, Total Carbohydrates: 0.5g, Dietary Fiber: 0g, Sugars: 0g, Protein: 6g*

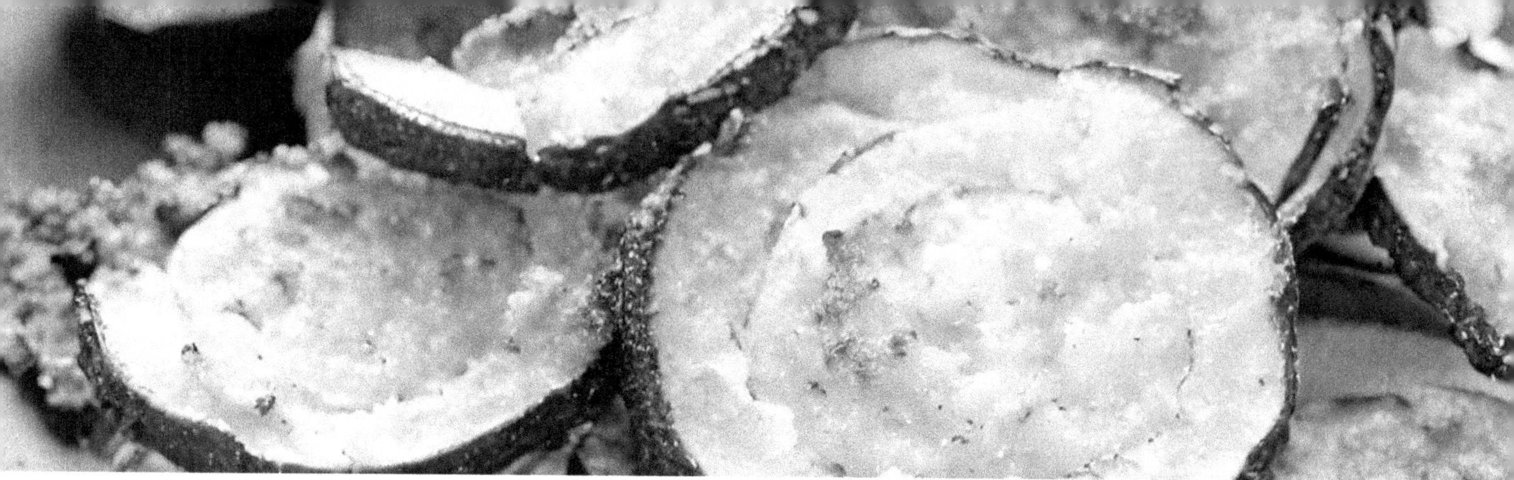

Zucchini Chips

INGREDIENTS

- 2 medium-sized zucchinis
- 2 tablespoons olive oil
- 1/4 teaspoon salt
- 1/4 teaspoon black pepper
- 1/4 teaspoon garlic powder (optional)
- 1/4 teaspoon paprika (optional)

INSTRUCTIONS

1. Preheat your oven to 425°F (220°C). Line a baking sheet with parchment paper to prevent sticking.

2. Wash the zucchinis and slice them into thin rounds, about 1/8 inch thick. Pat the zucchini slices dry with a paper towel to remove excess moisture.

3. In a mixing bowl, toss the zucchini slices with olive oil, salt, pepper, and any optional seasonings like garlic powder or paprika. Ensure that the zucchini slices are evenly coated.

4. Place the seasoned zucchini slices in a single layer on the prepared baking sheet. Make sure they are not overlapping to ensure even baking.

5. Place the baking sheet in the preheated oven and bake for 20-25 minutes or until the zucchini chips become golden brown and crispy. You may need to flip the chips halfway through the cooking time for even browning.

6. Remove the zucchini chips from the oven and let them cool on the baking sheet for a few minutes. They will become crispier as they cool down.

7. Transfer the zucchini chips to a serving plate and enjoy them as a low-carb snack.

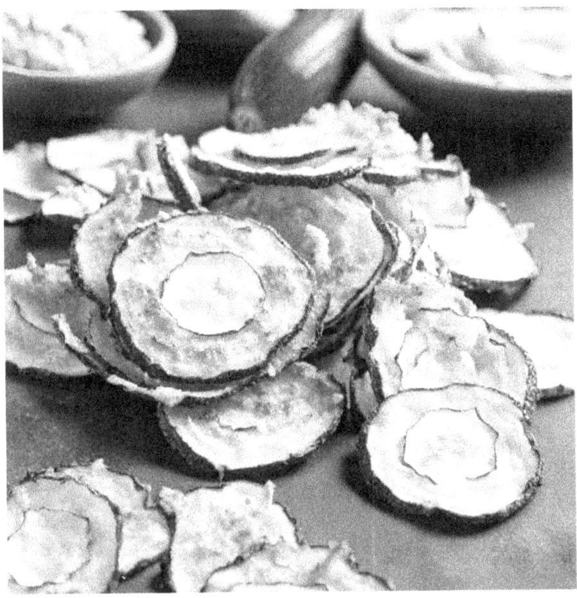

Tips for Variation:

- Experiment with different seasonings like grated Parmesan cheese, Italian herbs, or onion powder for unique flavors.
- Serve with a side of sugar-free marinara sauce for dipping.
- For a spicy kick, add a pinch of cayenne pepper or chili powder to the seasoning mix.
- Try making zucchini chips with a combination of yellow and green zucchinis for a colorful snack.

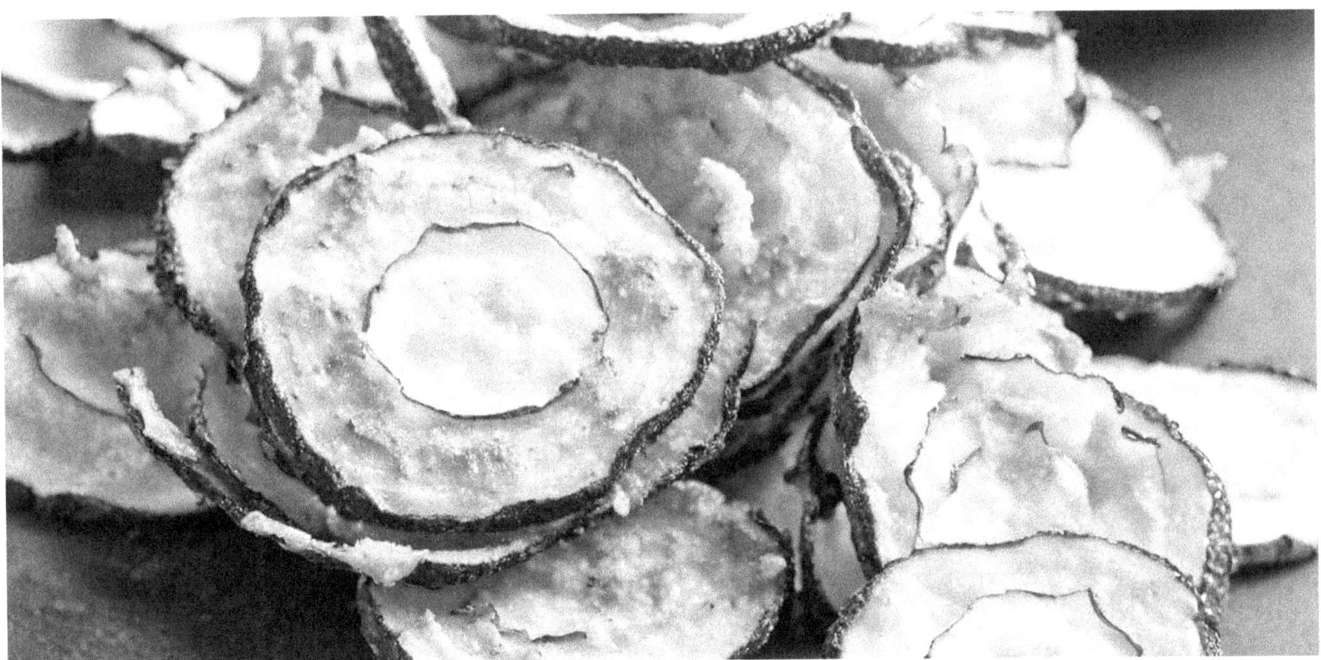

Nutritional Information: *Calories: 70 calories, Total Fat: 6g, Saturated Fat: 1g, Cholesterol: 0mg, Sodium: 150mg, Total Carbohydrates: 3g, Dietary Fiber: 1g, Sugars: 2g, Protein: 1g*

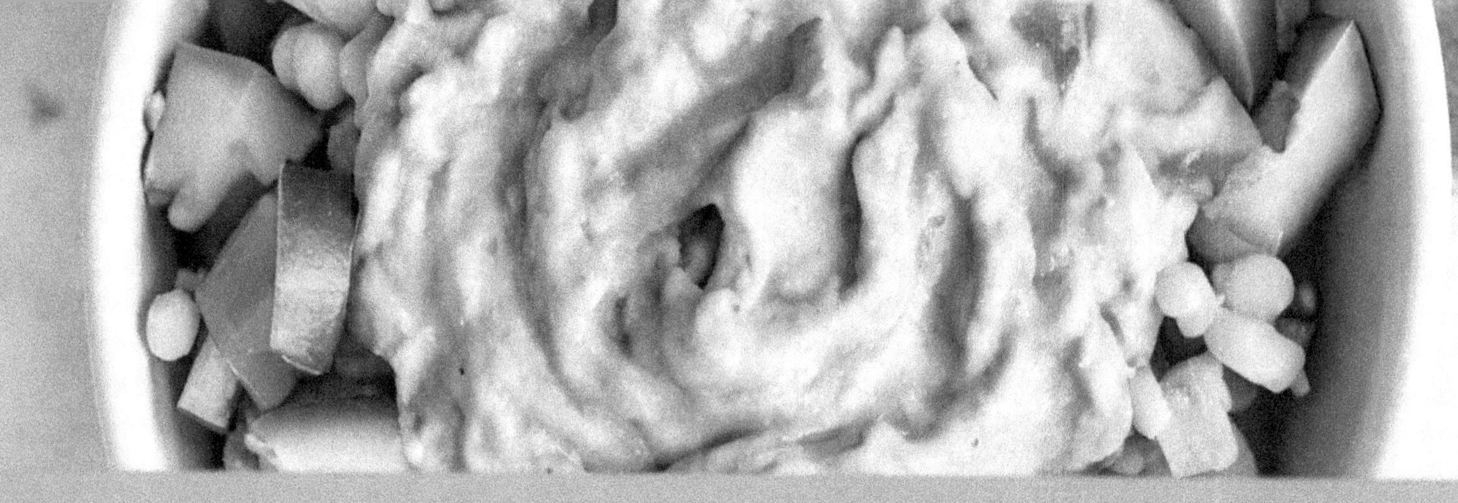

Guacamole with Veggies

SERVINGS: 4   PREP TIME: 15 MINUTES   COOK TIME: 0 MINUTES

INGREDIENTS

- 2 ripe avocados
- 1 small onion, finely chopped
- 1-2 cloves garlic, minced
- 1 small tomato, diced
- 1/4 cup fresh cilantro, chopped
- 1 jalapeño pepper, finely chopped (remove seeds for milder guacamole)
- Juice of 1 lime
- 1/2 teaspoon salt (adjust to taste)
- 1/4 teaspoon black pepper (optional)
- Assorted low-carb vegetables for dipping (e.g., cucumber slices, bell pepper strips, celery sticks)

INSTRUCTIONS

1. Cut the avocados in half, remove the pits, and scoop the flesh into a mixing bowl.

2. Use a fork to mash the avocados until you reach your desired level of creaminess. Some people prefer it chunky, while others prefer it smoother.

3. Add the finely chopped onion, minced garlic, diced tomato, chopped cilantro, and jalapeño pepper to the mashed avocados.

4. Squeeze the juice of one lime over the mixture. Add salt and pepper to taste. Gently stir all the ingredients together until well combined.

5. Taste the guacamole and adjust the seasonings if necessary. You can add more lime juice, salt, or pepper according to your preference.

6. Ensure it touches the surface to prevent browning. Refrigerate for at least 30 minutes to allow the flavors to meld.

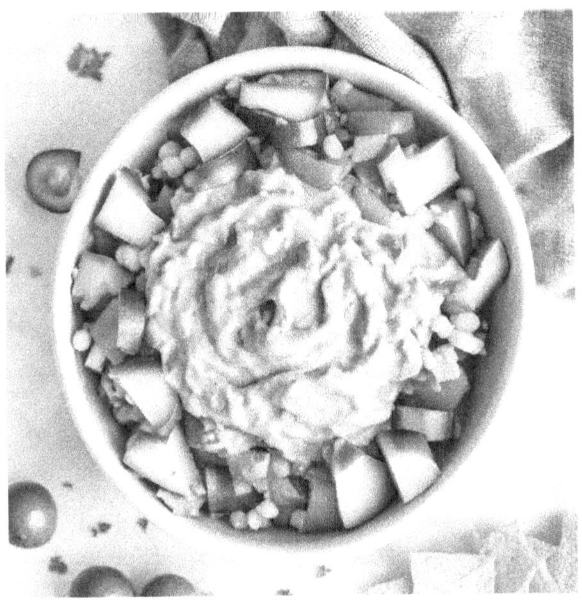

7. Serve the guacamole in a bowl alongside a platter of low-carb vegetables for dipping.

Tips for Variation:

- Customize the level of spiciness by adjusting the amount of jalapeño pepper.
- Add diced bell peppers, diced cucumber, or diced red onion for added texture and flavor.
- For a creamy twist, mix in a tablespoon of sour cream or Greek yogurt.
- Sprinkle crumbled feta cheese or cotija cheese on top for a savory touch.
- Consider adding a dash of cayenne pepper or chili powder for extra heat.

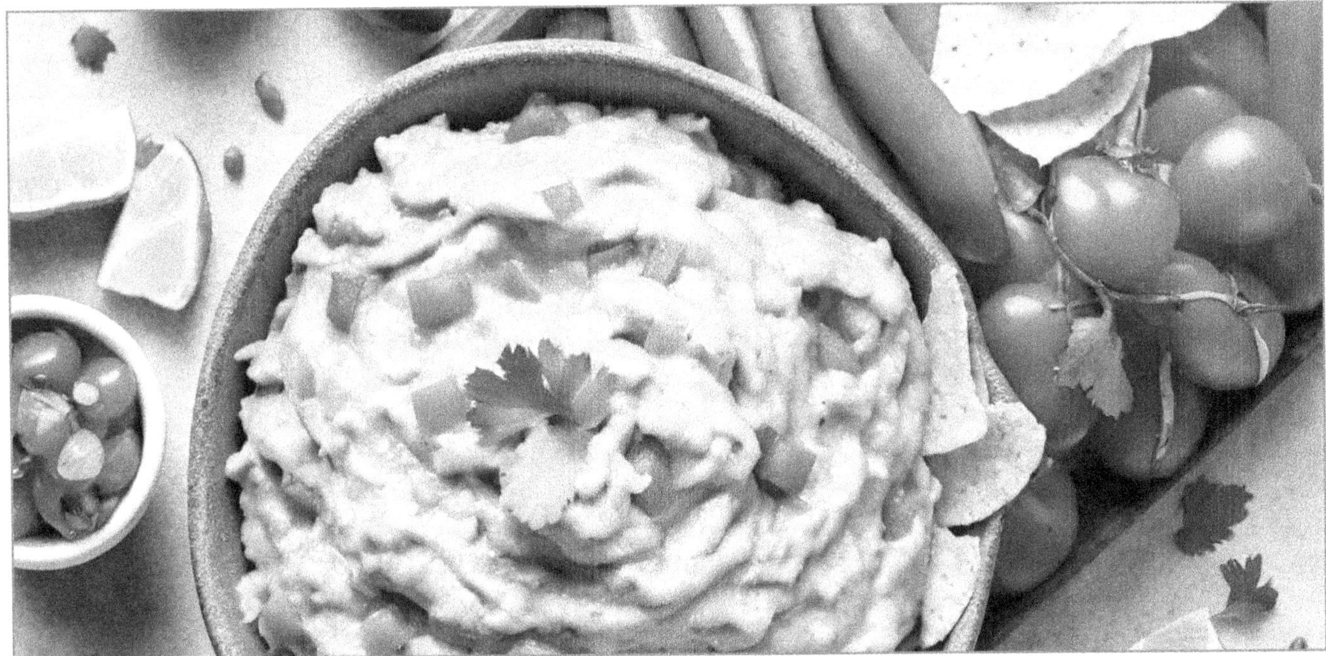

Nutritional Information: *Calories: 160 calories, Total Fat: 14g, Saturated Fat: 2g, Cholesterol: 0mg, Sodium: 300mg, Total Carbohydrates: 10g, Dietary Fiber: 7g, Sugars: 2g, Protein: 2g*

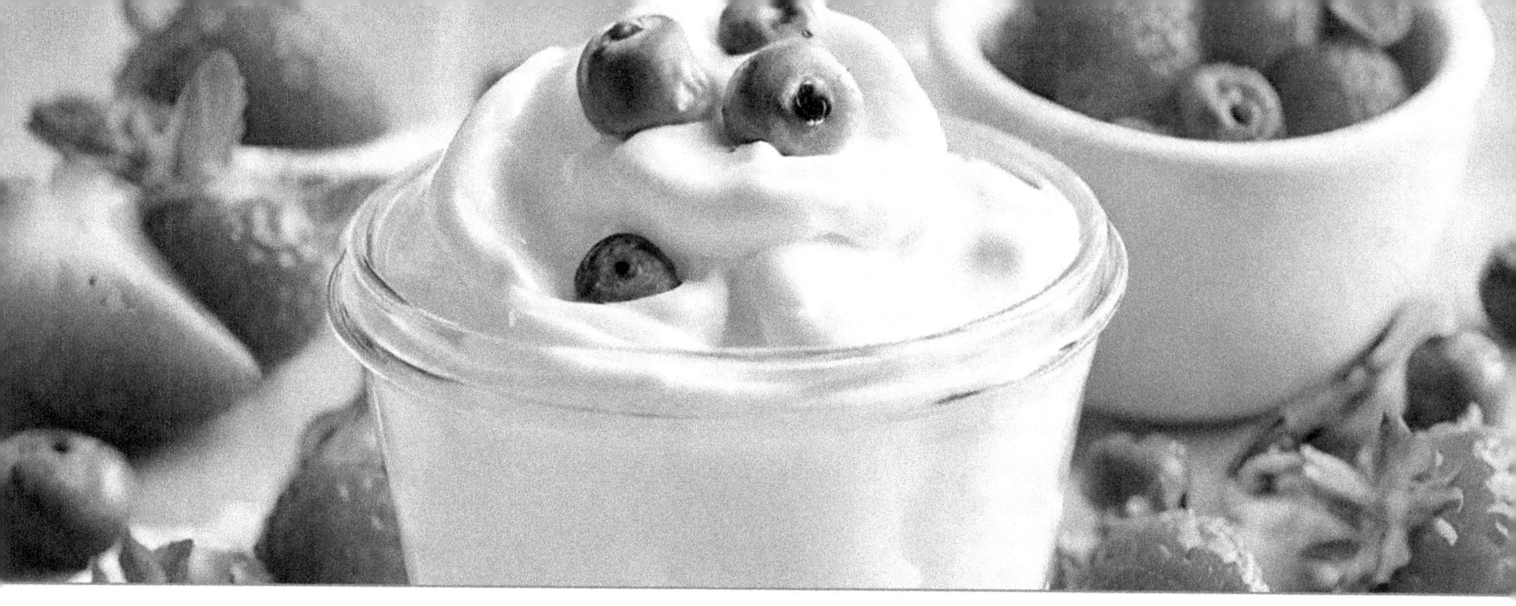

Greek Yogurt Parfait

INGREDIENTS

- 1 cup plain Greek yogurt (full-fat or low-fat, according to your preference)
- 1/2 cup mixed berries (e.g., strawberries, blueberries, raspberries)
- 1/4 cup chopped nuts (e.g., almonds, walnuts, pecans)
- 1 tablespoon sugar-free sweetener (e.g., stevia, erythritol) (optional)
- 1/2 teaspoon vanilla extract (optional)

INSTRUCTIONS

1. If you'd like, you can add a sweetener and vanilla extract to the Greek yogurt for added flavor. Mix well.

2. Use a clear glass or a small bowl to create layers of yogurt, berries, and nuts. Start with a spoonful of Greek yogurt at the bottom.

3. Add a layer of mixed berries on top of the yogurt. You can use a combination of your favorite low-carb berries.

4. Continue layering with another spoonful of yogurt and more berries until you've used up your ingredients. Finish with a final layer of yogurt on top.

5. Sprinkle the chopped nuts over the yogurt parfait. They add crunch, flavor, and healthy fats.

6. If desired, garnish with an extra berry or a small mint leaf for a visually appealing touch.

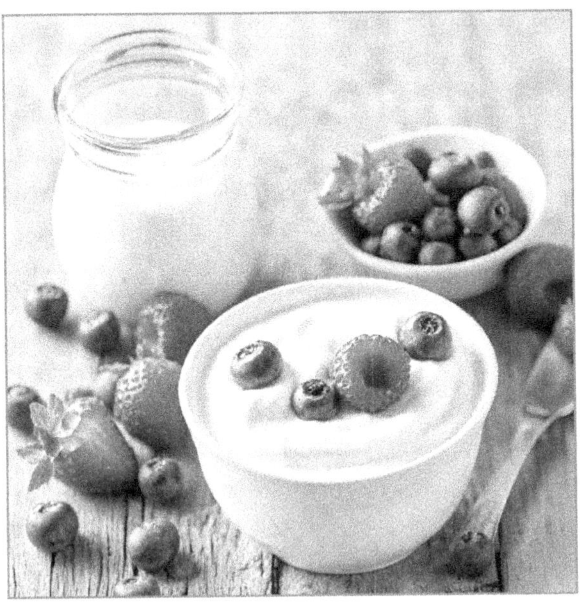

7. Enjoy your Greek Yogurt Parfait immediately or refrigerate until you're ready to eat.

Tips for Variation:

- Experiment with different flavors of Greek yogurt, such as vanilla or coconut-flavored.

- Use a variety of low-carb fruits like sliced peaches, cherries, or blackberries.

- Add a drizzle of sugar-free chocolate or caramel sauce for extra indulgence.

- For extra crunch, sprinkle a tablespoon of granola or crushed low-carb nuts and seeds.

- If you're not concerned about carbs, you can add a tablespoon of chia seeds for added fiber and texture.

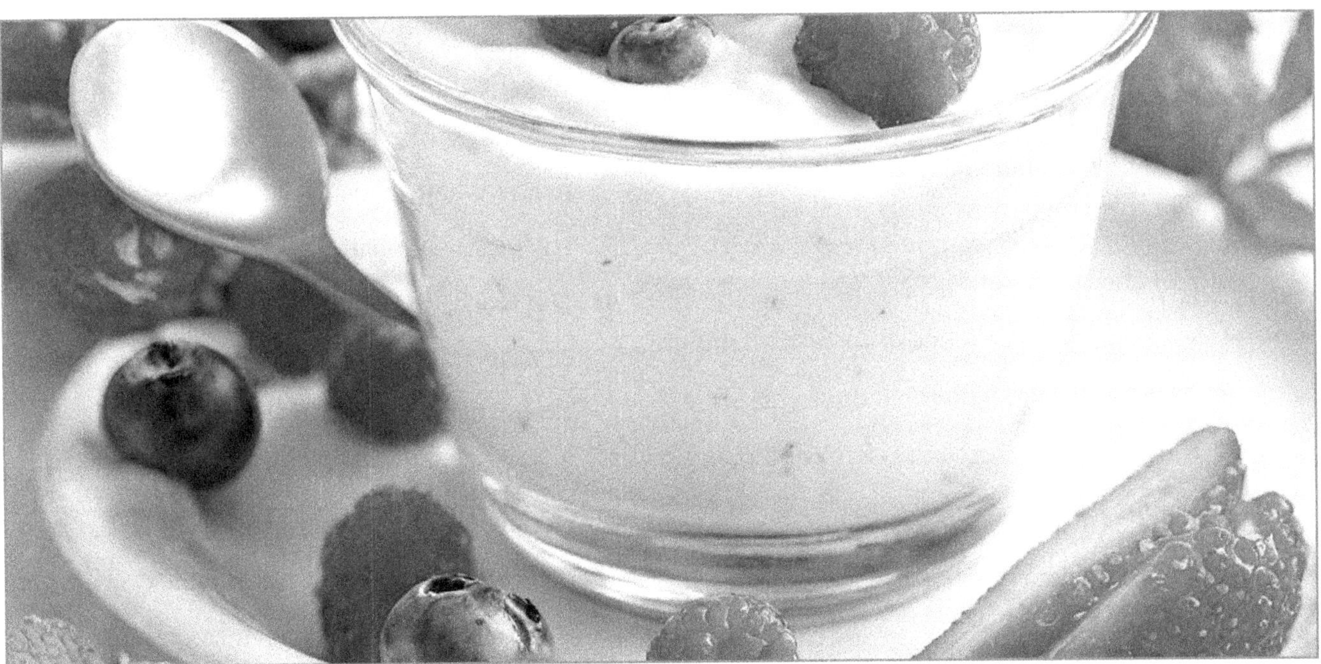

Nutritional Information: *Calories: 350 calories, Total Fat: 20g, Saturated Fat: 2g, Cholesterol: 10mg, Sodium: 50mg, Total Carbohydrates: 23g, Dietary Fiber: 6g, Sugars: 12g (from natural sugars in the berries, not added sugars), Protein: 24g*

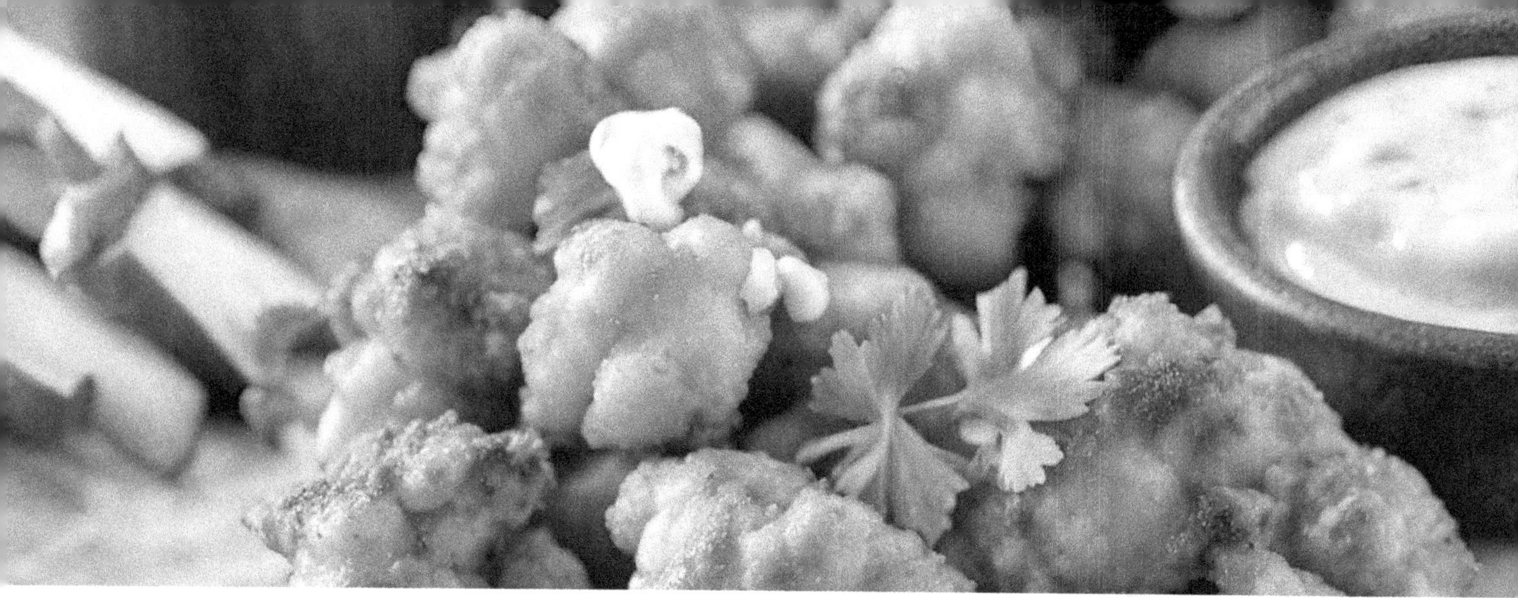

Buffalo Cauliflower Bites

INGREDIENTS

- 1 medium head of cauliflower, cut into bite-sized florets
- 1/2 cup almond flour
- 1/2 cup unsweetened almond milk (or any low-carb milk of your choice)
- 1/2 teaspoon garlic powder
- 1/2 teaspoon onion powder
- 1/4 teaspoon paprika
- Salt and black pepper to taste
- 1/4 cup hot sauce (choose a low-carb option)
- 2 tablespoons unsalted butter or ghee
- Ranch or blue cheese dressing for dipping (optional)
- Chopped celery and carrot sticks for serving (optional)

INSTRUCTIONS

1. Preheat your oven to 450°F (230°C). Line a baking sheet with parchment paper for easy cleanup.

2. Cut the cauliflower into bite-sized florets. Rinse them and pat them dry with paper towels.

3. In a mixing bowl, combine the almond flour, almond milk, garlic powder, onion powder, paprika, salt, and black pepper. Stir until you have a smooth batter.

4. Dip each cauliflower floret into the batter, ensuring it's evenly coated. Shake off any excess batter.

5. Arrange the coated cauliflower on the prepared baking sheet in a single layer. Bake in the preheated oven for 20-25 minutes or until the cauliflower is tender and the coating becomes crispy, flipping them halfway through.

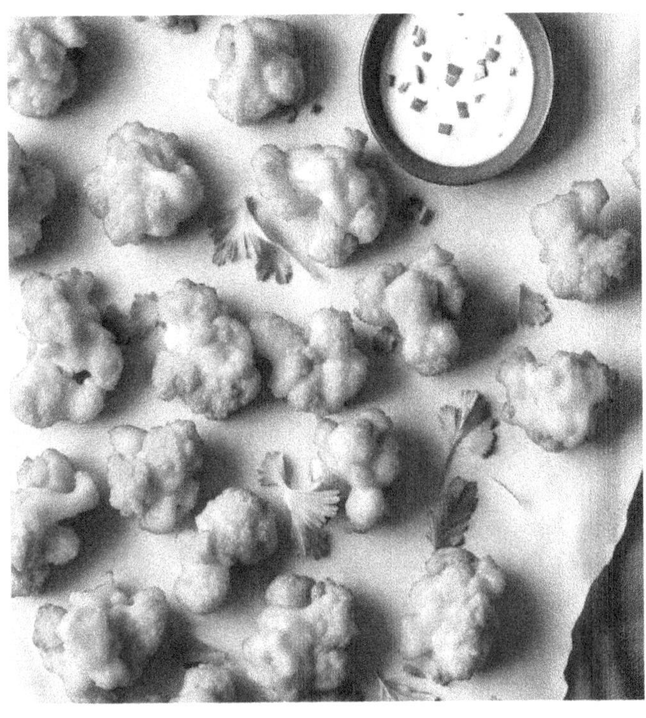

6. While the cauliflower is baking, in a small saucepan, melt the butter over low heat. Stir in the hot sauce and cook for a few minutes until well combined. Adjust the level of spiciness to your liking.

7. Once the cauliflower is done baking, remove it from the oven. Transfer the cauliflower to a mixing bowl, pour the buffalo sauce over it, and gently toss to coat the cauliflower evenly with the sauce.

8. Serve the Buffalo Cauliflower Bites hot with a side of ranch or blue cheese dressing and optional celery and carrot sticks for dipping.

<u>Tips for Variation:</u>

- Adjust the level of spiciness by using more or less hot sauce in the buffalo sauce mixture.
- For a crispy coating, consider adding a tablespoon of grated Parmesan cheese to the almond flour mixture.
- If you prefer a milder version, you can use BBQ sauce or a mixture of melted butter and garlic instead of buffalo sauce.
- Serve with a side of celery and carrot sticks for a refreshing crunch and added nutrients.

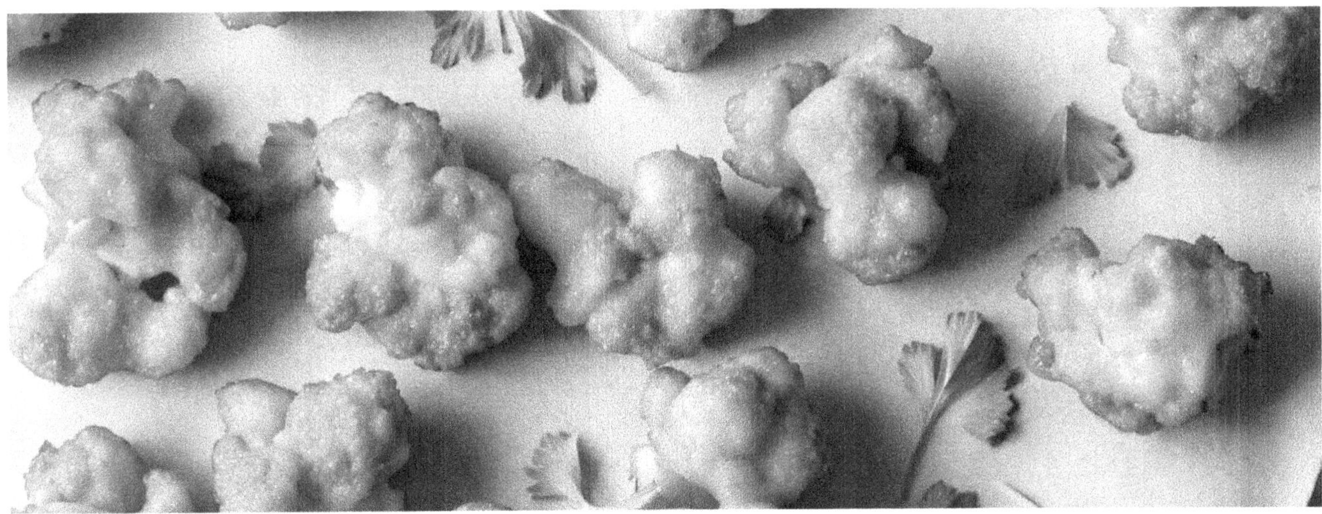

<u>Nutritional Information:</u> *Calories: 190 calories, Total Fat: 14g, Saturated Fat: 5g, Cholesterol: 20mg, Sodium: 540mg, Total Carbohydrates: 8g, Dietary Fiber: 4g, Sugars: 2g, Protein: 6g*

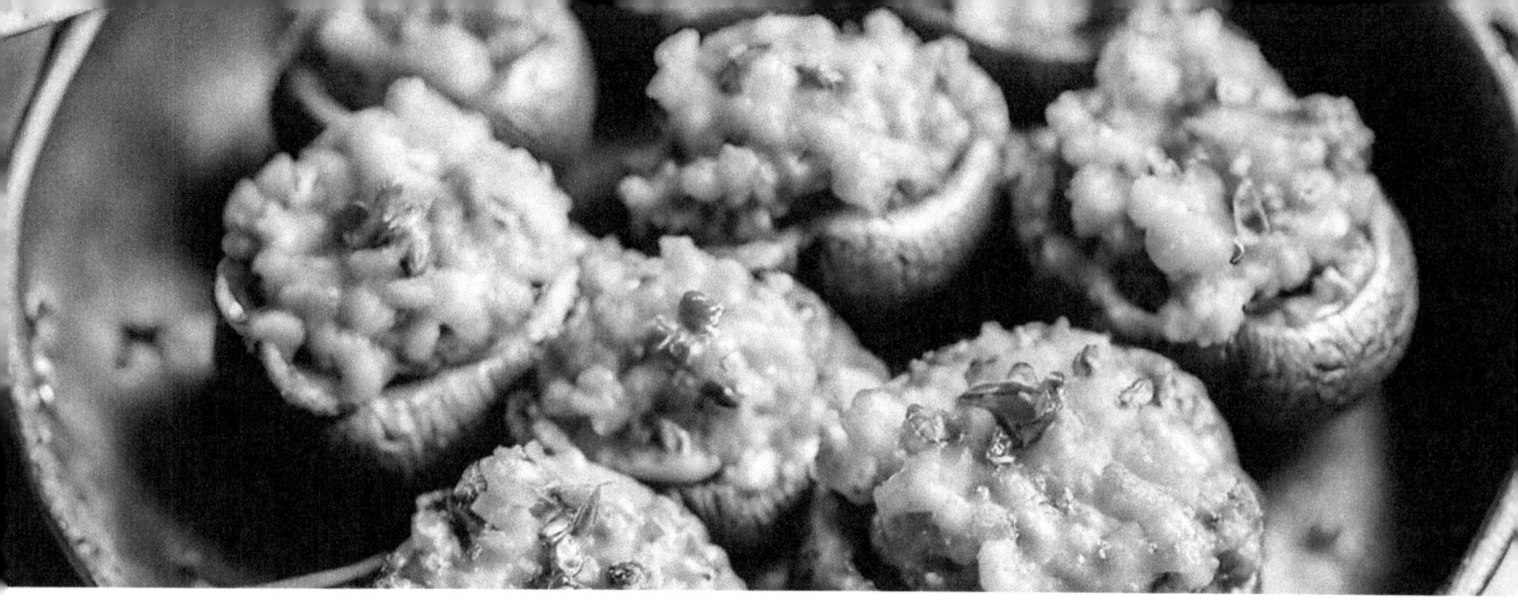

Stuffed Mushrooms

SERVINGS: 12   PREP TIME: 20 MINUTES   COOK TIME: 20 To 25 MINUTES

INGREDIENTS

- 12 large mushrooms (about 2 inches in diameter)
- 8 oz. (225g) cream cheese, softened
- 1/4 cup grated Parmesan cheese
- 2 cloves garlic, minced
- 2 tablespoons fresh parsley, finely chopped
- 1/4 teaspoon black pepper
- 1/4 teaspoon onion powder
- 1/4 teaspoon dried oregano
- 1/4 teaspoon dried thyme
- 1/4 teaspoon dried basil
- Salt to taste
- 2 tablespoons olive oil
- Chopped fresh parsley for garnish (optional)

INSTRUCTIONS

1. Preheat your oven to 375°F (190°C).
2. Clean the mushrooms by gently wiping them with a damp paper towel to remove any dirt. Carefully remove the stems from the mushrooms, leaving the caps intact. Set the mushroom caps aside.
3. In a mixing bowl, combine the softened cream cheese, grated Parmesan cheese, minced garlic, chopped parsley, black pepper, onion powder, dried oregano, dried thyme, dried basil, and a pinch of salt. Mix until all the ingredients are well incorporated.
4. Using a small spoon or your fingers, fill each mushroom cap with the cream cheese mixture, making sure to pack it down gently and create a mound on top.
5. Place the stuffed mushrooms on a baking sheet lined with parchment paper to prevent sticking.

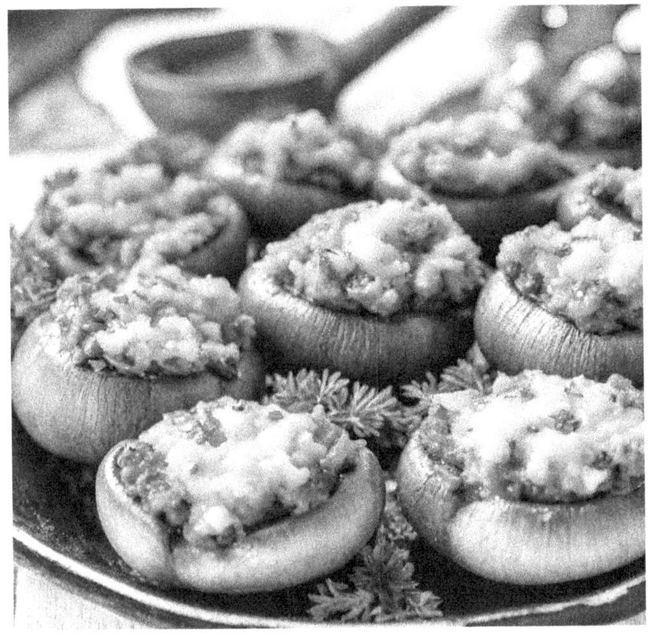

6. Drizzle the olive oil evenly over the stuffed mushrooms.

7. Bake in the preheated oven for approximately 20-25 minutes or until the mushrooms are tender and the filling is golden brown and slightly crispy on top.

8. If desired, garnish the stuffed mushrooms with chopped fresh parsley before serving.

9. Serve the Stuffed Mushrooms hot as a delicious appetizer or snack.

Tips for Variation:

- Add finely chopped cooked bacon or cooked sausage to the cream cheese mixture for added flavor and protein.

- Experiment with different herbs and spices in the filling, such as dill, rosemary, or chili flakes, to suit your taste.

- Top each stuffed mushroom with a small slice of mozzarella or cheddar cheese for a cheesy twist.

- For a vegetarian version, omit the Parmesan cheese and use a dairy-free cream cheese substitute.

- Serve with a low-carb marinara sauce or ranch dressing for dipping.

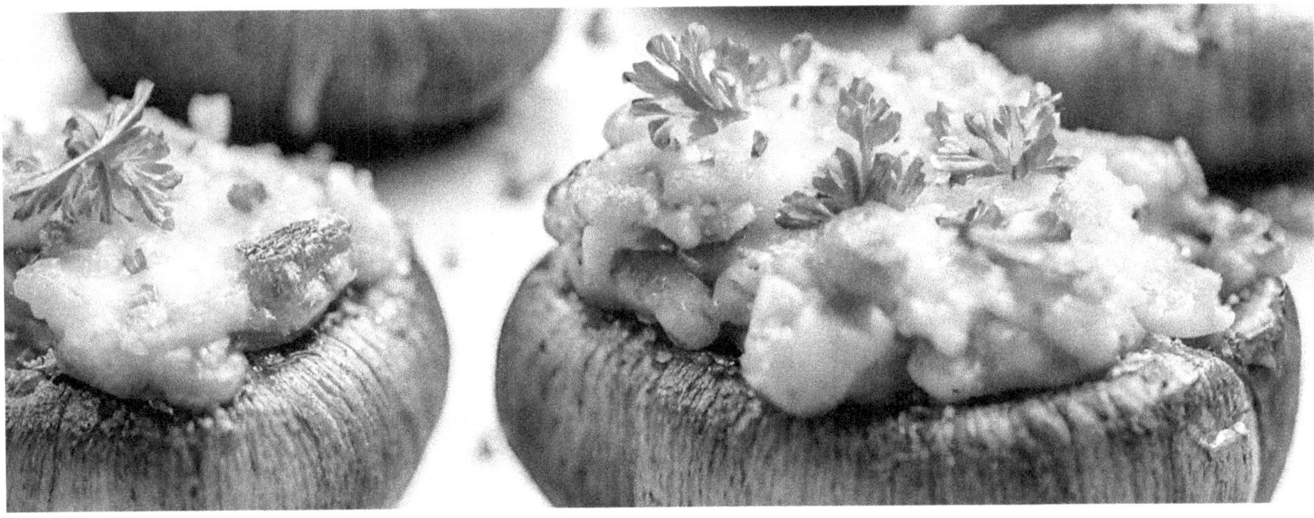

Nutritional Information: *Calories: 200 calories, Total Fat: 18g, Saturated Fat: 8g, Cholesterol: 40mg, Sodium: 250mg, Total Carbohydrates: 4g, Dietary Fiber: 1g, Sugars: 2g, Protein: 6g*

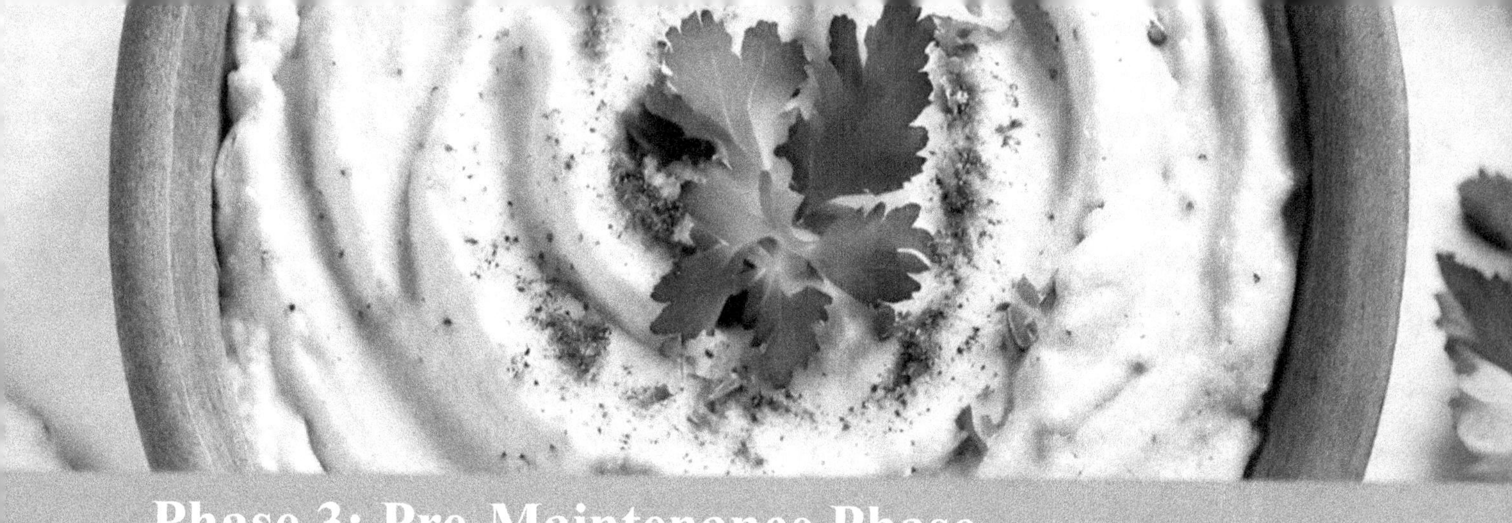

Cauliflower Hummus

SERVINGS: 8   PREP TIME: 15 MINUTES   COOK TIME: 10 TO 12 MINUTES

INGREDIENTS

- 1 medium cauliflower head, cut into florets (about 4 cups)
- 3 tablespoons tahini (sesame paste)
- 2 cloves garlic, minced
- 3 tablespoons olive oil
- Juice of 1 lemon
- 1/2 teaspoon ground cumin
- 1/2 teaspoon paprika
- 1/4 teaspoon salt (adjust to taste)
- 1/4 teaspoon black pepper
- 2 tablespoons chopped fresh parsley (for garnish)
- Extra olive oil and paprika for drizzling (optional)

INSTRUCTIONS

1. Steam the cauliflower florets until they are very tender, about 10-12 minutes. Alternatively, you can boil them in water until fork-tender. Drain and let cool slightly.

2. In a food processor, combine the cooked cauliflower, tahini, minced garlic, olive oil, lemon juice, ground cumin, paprika, salt, and black pepper.

3. Process the ingredients until you achieve a smooth and creamy consistency. You may need to scrape down the sides of the food processor and blend again to ensure all the ingredients are well incorporated.

4. Taste the cauliflower hummus and adjust the seasonings to your liking. You can add more lemon juice, salt, or spices if desired.

5. Transfer the cauliflower hummus to a serving bowl, cover, and refrigerate for at least 30 minutes to allow the flavors to meld.

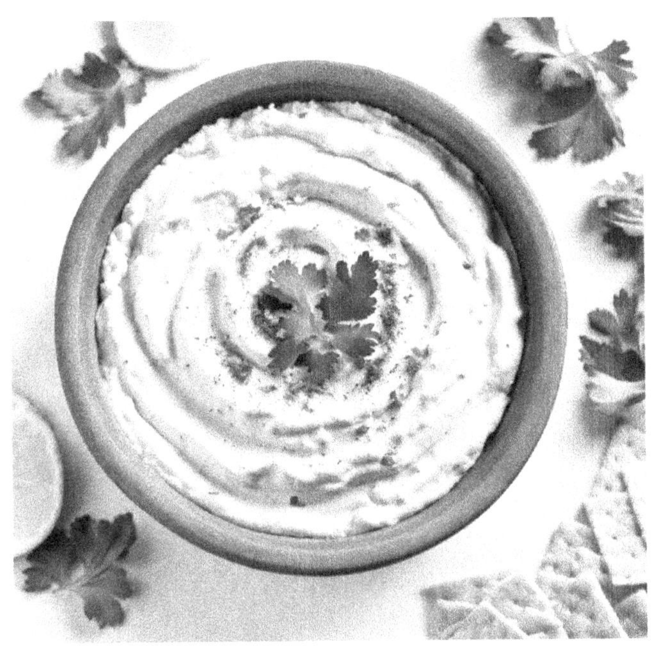

6. Before serving, garnish the cauliflower hummus with chopped fresh parsley. If desired, drizzle with extra olive oil and sprinkle with a dash of paprika for added flavor and presentation.

7. Serve the Cauliflower Hummus with your favorite low-carb dippers, such as cucumber slices, bell pepper strips, or celery sticks.

Tips for Variation:

- Add roasted red pepper or sun-dried tomatoes for a different flavor profile.

- Include a pinch of smoked paprika or cayenne pepper for a smoky or spicy kick.

- Top with pine nuts, toasted sesame seeds, or a drizzle of balsamic reduction for texture and flavor.

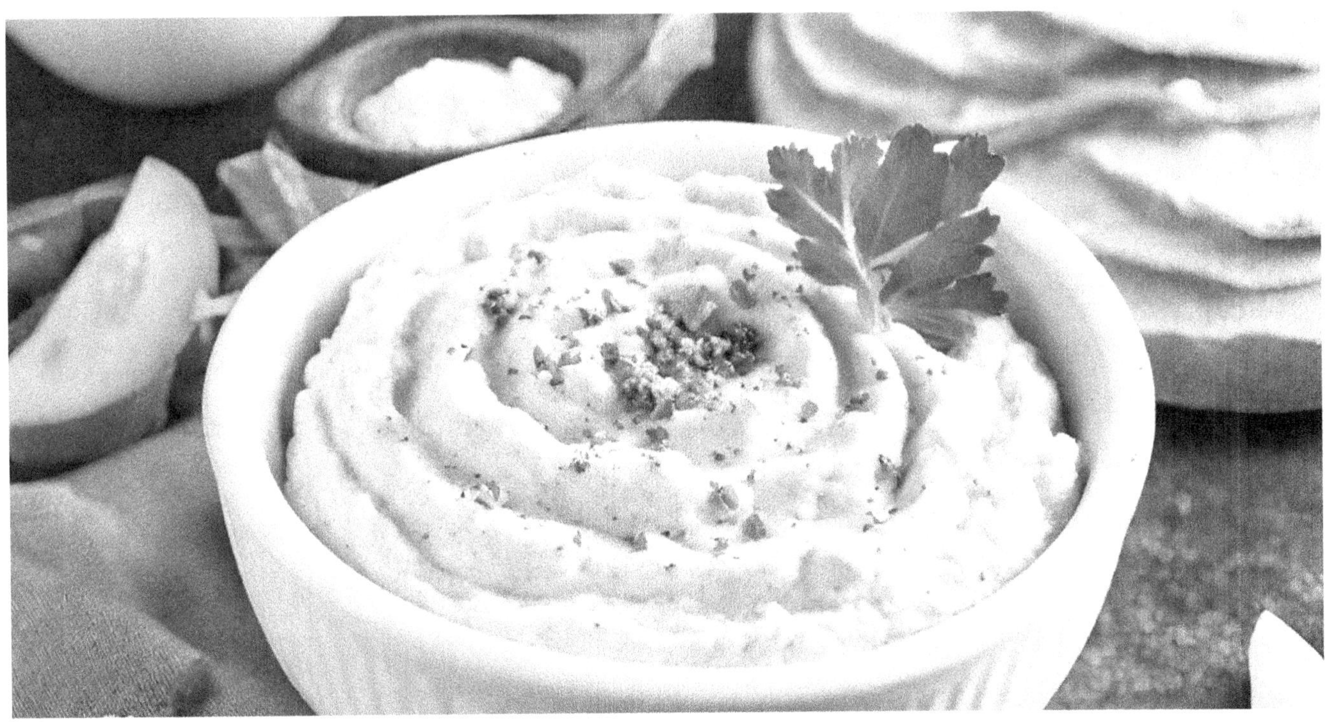

Nutritional Information: *Calories: 100 calories, Total Fat: 8g, Saturated Fat: 1g, Cholesterol: 0mg, Sodium: 120mg, Total Carbohydrates: 5g, Dietary Fiber: 2g, Sugars: 1g, Protein: 2g*

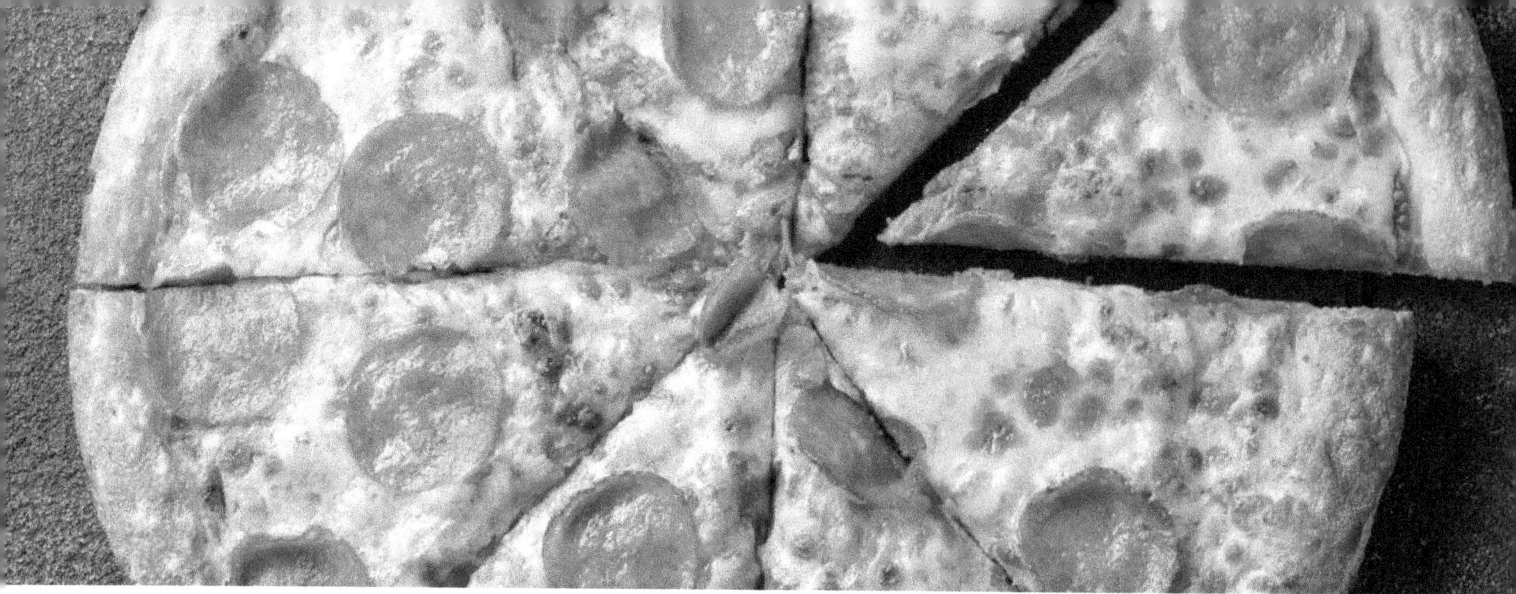

Cheese and Pepperoni

INGREDIENTS

- 12 slices of pepperoni (look for a brand with low or no added sugar)
- 4 oz. (about 1 cup) of your favorite low-carb cheese, such as mozzarella, cheddar, or Swiss
- 1 tablespoon olive oil (optional, for dipping)
- Red pepper flakes (optional, for added spice)

<u>Tips for Variation:</u>

- Customize your cheese selection with options like provolone, Gouda, or pepper jack for different flavors.
- Add a variety of low-carb vegetables, such as cherry tomatoes, cucumber slices, or olives, to create a keto-friendly charcuterie board.
- For a spicy kick, try using jalapeño or pepper jack cheese and using spicy pepperoni slices.

INSTRUCTIONS

1. Cut the cheese into bite-sized cubes, sticks, or slices, depending on your preference. You can mix and match different types of low-carb cheeses for variety.
2. Arrange the cheese and pepperoni on a serving platter or plate. You can alternate between cheese and pepperoni slices for a visually appealing presentation.
3. If desired, you can provide a small bowl of olive oil for dipping the cheese or drizzling it over the pepperoni. You can also sprinkle red pepper flakes for added spice.
4. Serve the Cheese and Pepperoni as a delicious and satisfying low-carb snack or appetizer.

<u>**Nutritional Information:**</u> *Calories: 220 calories, Total Fat: 18g, Saturated Fat: 9g, Cholesterol: 45mg, Sodium: 420mg, Total Carbohydrates: 1g, Dietary Fiber: 0g, Sugars: 0g, Protein: 13g*

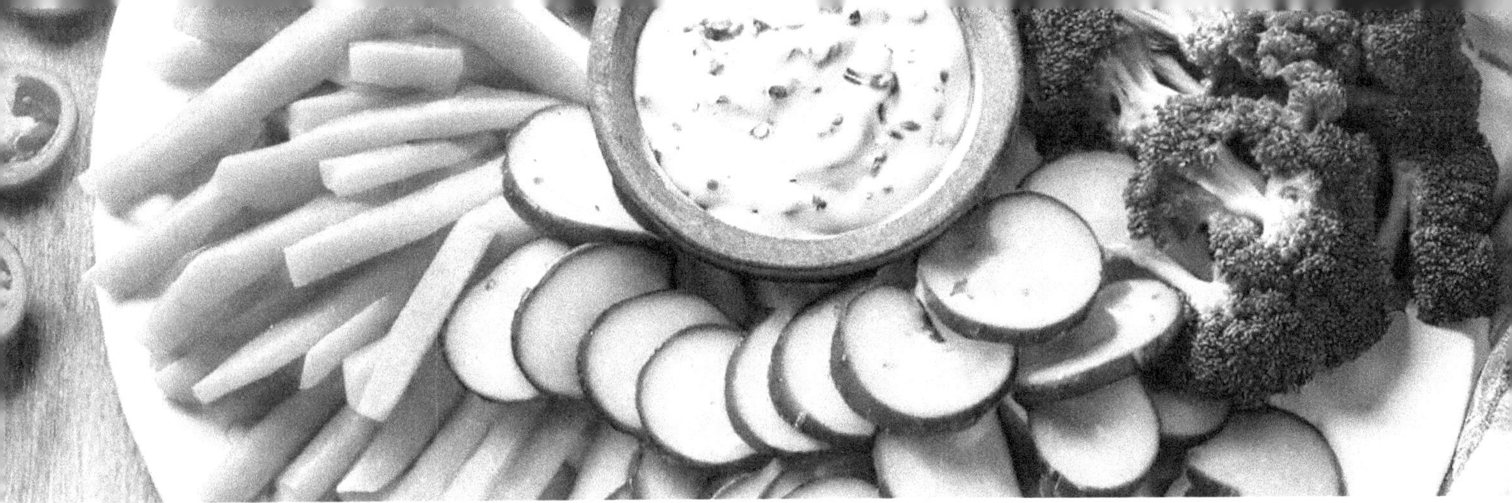

Sliced Veggies with Ranch Dressing

SERVINGS: 2   PREP TIME: 10 MINUTES   COOK TIME: 0 MINUTE

- 2 cups of mixed low-carb vegetables (e.g., cucumber slices, bell pepper strips, celery sticks, cherry tomatoes, and broccoli florets)
- 1/4 cup sugar-free ranch dressing (store-bought or homemade)
- Fresh herbs for garnish (optional, e.g., chopped fresh parsley or dill)

Tips for Variation:

- Add some radishes, jicama sticks, or cauliflower florets for additional variety in your veggie platter.
- Make your own homemade low-carb ranch dressing using mayonnaise, sour cream, buttermilk (or a low-carb substitute), and a mix of herbs and spices.

1. Wash and slice the low-carb vegetables into bite-sized pieces or strips. You can choose your favorite low-carb vegetables, such as cucumbers, bell peppers, celery, cherry tomatoes, and broccoli.
2. Arrange the sliced vegetables on a serving platter or in a bowl. You can arrange them in a visually appealing pattern.
3. Place the sugar-free ranch dressing in a small bowl or ramekin, and set it alongside the sliced vegetables.
4. If desired, garnish the dish with fresh herbs like chopped parsley or dill for added freshness and presentation.
5. Serve the Sliced Veggies with Ranch Dressing as a delightful low-carb snack or appetizer.

Nutritional Information: *(per serving): Calories: 120 calories, Total Fat: 10g, Saturated Fat: 2g, Cholesterol: 10mg, Sodium: 300mg, Total Carbohydrates: 6g, Dietary Fiber: 2g, Sugars: 3g, Protein: 2g*

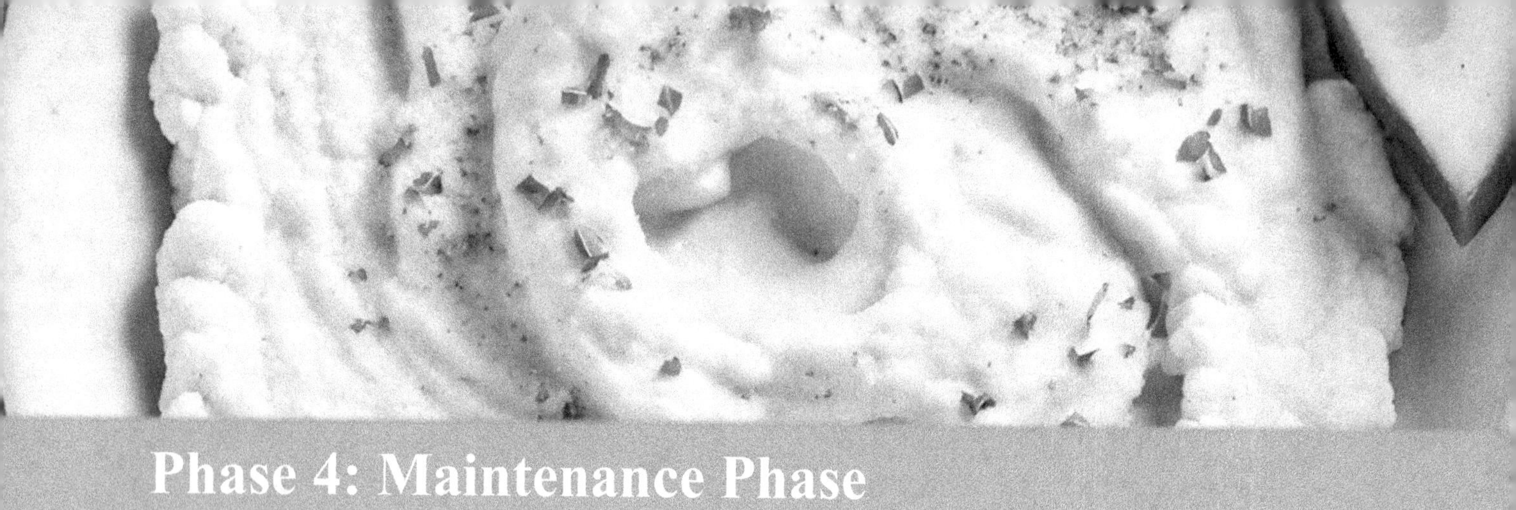

Almond Butter and Celery

SERVINGS: 2   PREP TIME: 5 MINUTES   COOK TIME: 0 MINUTE

INGREDIENTS

- 2 stalks of celery, washed and trimmed
- 2 tablespoons almond butter (sugar-free and unsweetened)

INSTRUCTIONS

1. Cut the celery stalks into manageable lengths, typically about 4 to 5 inches long.
2. Use a knife to spread almond butter onto each celery stalk. You can spread it generously, adjusting to your preference.
3. Arrange the almond butter-filled celery stalks on a plate and serve as a nutritious and satisfying snack.

Tips for Variation:

- You can use other nut or seed butters like peanut butter, cashew butter, or sunflower seed butter if you prefer.
- Add a sprinkle of cinnamon or a drizzle of sugar-free syrup on top for extra flavor.
- For a crunchy twist, sprinkle some chopped nuts or seeds on the almond butter.
- Experiment with different veggies like cucumber or bell pepper strips as an alternative to celery.

Nutritional Information (per serving): *Calories: 120 calories, Total Fat: 10g, Saturated Fat: 1g, Cholesterol: 0mg, Sodium: 60mg, Total Carbohydrates: 5g, Dietary Fiber: 2g, Sugars: 2g, Protein: 3g*

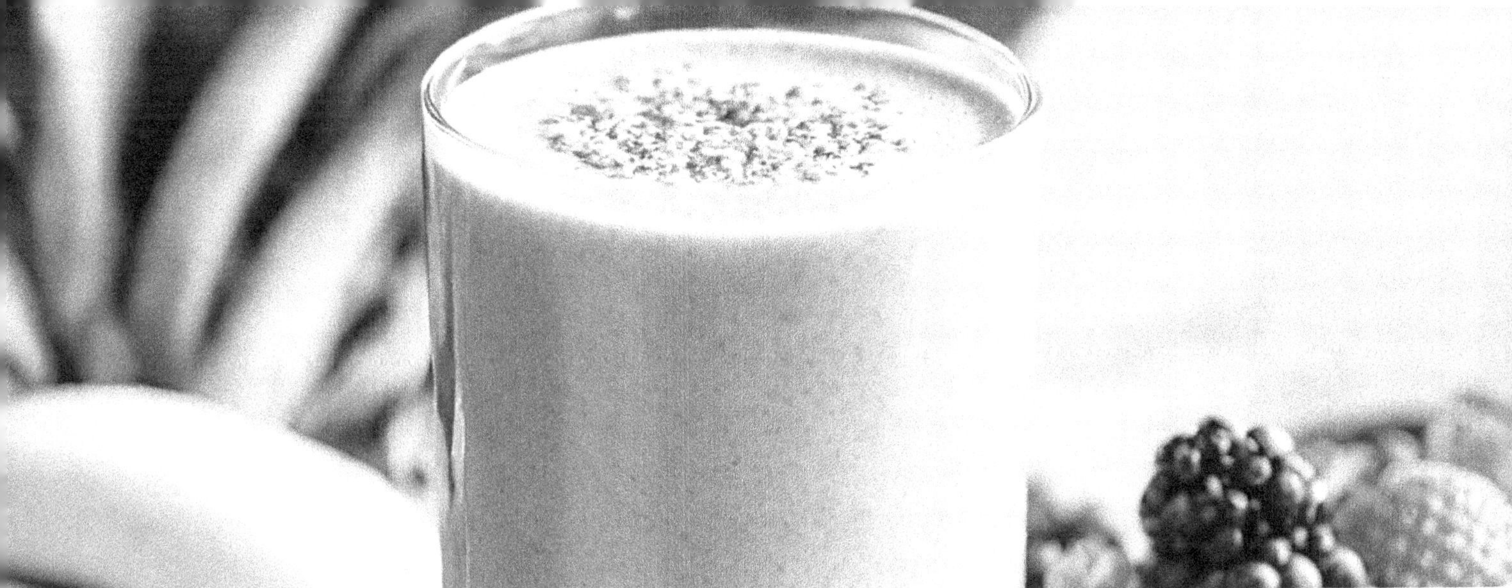

Protein Smoothie

- 1 cup unsweetened almond milk or other low-carb milk
- 1 scoop of low-carb protein powder (vanilla or chocolate flavor)
- 1 tablespoon almond butter (sugar-free and unsweetened)
- 1/2 cup frozen mixed berries (e.g., strawberries, blueberries, raspberries)
- 1/2 cup baby spinach leaves (optional)
- Ice cubes (optional, for thickness)
- Sweetener (e.g., stevia or erythritol) to taste (optional)

1. In a blender, add almond milk, protein powder, almond butter, frozen berries, baby spinach (if using), and ice cubes (if desired).
2. Blend all the ingredients until you achieve a smooth and creamy consistency. If you'd like a thicker smoothie, add more ice cubes or reduce the amount of almond milk.
3. Taste the smoothie and add a sweetener of your choice, such as stevia or erythritol, if desired. Blend briefly to combine.
4. Pour the Protein Smoothie into a glass and enjoy immediately as a protein-packed snack.

Tips for Variation:

- Customize your smoothie by adding other low-carb ingredients like chia seeds, flax seeds, or a handful of your favorite low-carb berries.

Nutritional Information (per serving): Calories: 250 calories, Total Fat: 11g, Saturated Fat: 1g, Cholesterol: 15mg, Sodium: 400mg, Total Carbohydrates: 12g, Dietary Fiber: 6g, Sugars: 2g, Protein:

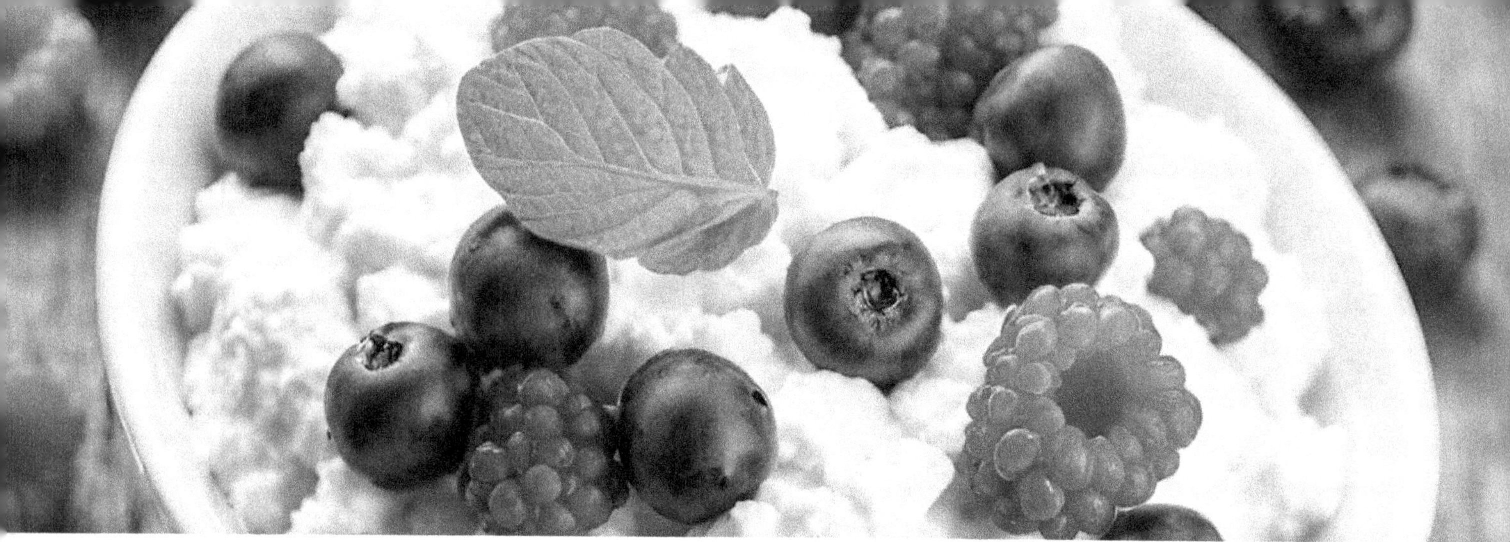

Cottage Cheese with Berries

INGREDIENTS

- 1 cup full-fat cottage cheese
- 1/2 cup mixed berries (e.g., strawberries, blueberries, raspberries)
- 1 tablespoon sugar-free sweetener (e.g., stevia or erythritol) (optional)
- 1/4 teaspoon vanilla extract (optional)
- Fresh mint leaves for garnish (optional)

Tips for Variation:

- Experiment with different low-carb fruits, such as blackberries, cherries, or sliced peaches, to change up the flavor profile.
- Add a handful of chopped nuts (e.g., almonds or walnuts) for extra crunch and healthy fats.
- Drizzle a small amount of sugar-free chocolate sauce or caramel sauce for a decadent twist.

INSTRUCTIONS

1. Wash and prepare the mixed berries. You can slice strawberries and leave smaller berries like blueberries and raspberries whole.

2. If desired, sprinkle the sugar-free sweetener over the berries and gently toss them to sweeten. Adjust the amount of sweetener to your taste.

3. In a serving bowl, scoop out the full-fat cottage cheese.

4. For added flavor, you can stir in the vanilla extract into the cottage cheese.

5. Arrange the sweetened mixed berries on top of the cottage cheese.

6. If desired, garnish the dish with fresh mint leaves for a touch of freshness and presentation.

7. Serve the Cottage Cheese with Berries as a delicious and satisfying snack or dessert.

Nutritional Information (per serving): *Calories: 280 calories, Total Fat: 11g, Saturated Fat: 6g, Cholesterol: 40mg, Sodium: 700mg, Total Carbohydrates: 16g, Dietary Fiber: 4g, Sugars: 8g, Protein: 28g*

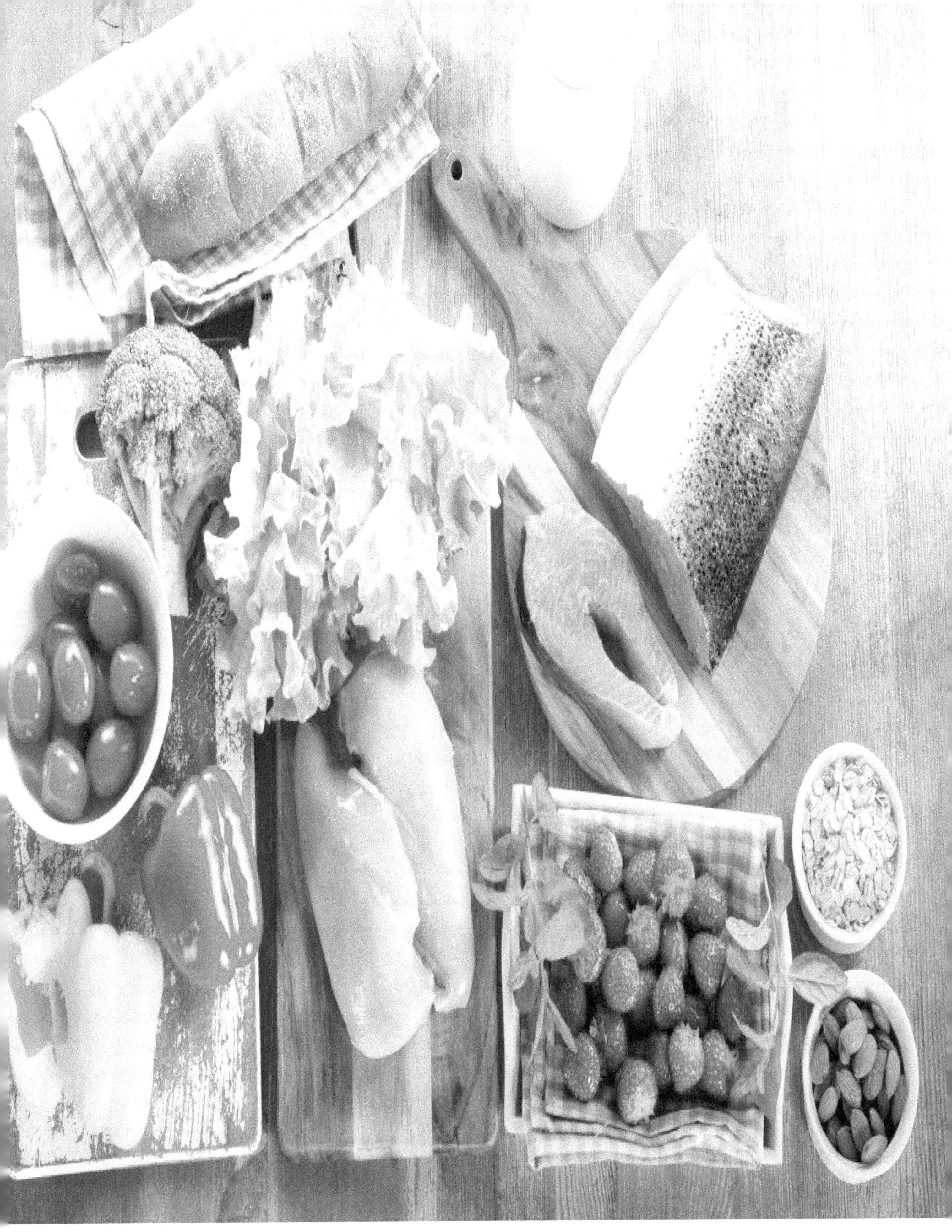

Notes:

Your
Observation:

Progress
Report:

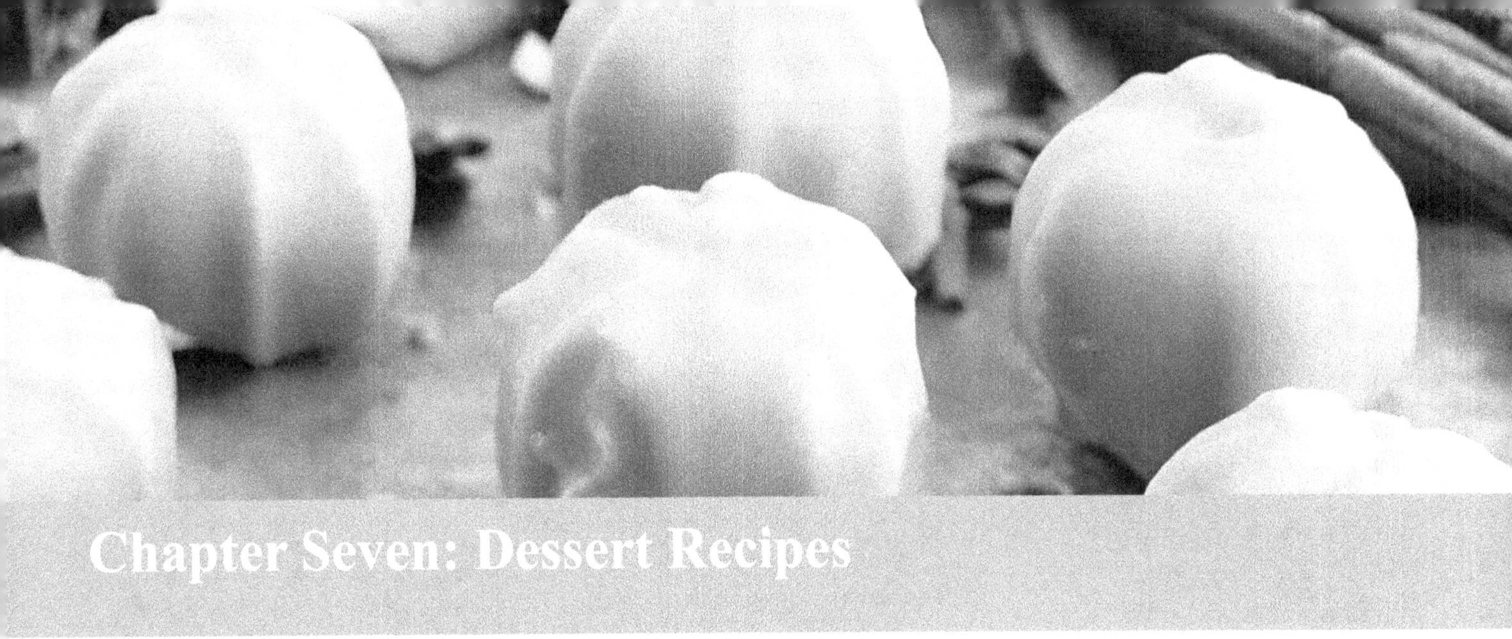

Phase 1: Induction Recipes

Pumpkin Spice Fat Bombs

SERVINGS: 4 FAT BOMBS   PREP TIME: 10 MINUTES   COOK TIME: 0 MINUTES

- 1/2 cup canned pumpkin puree (unsweetened)
- 1/2 cup coconut oil, melted
- 2 tablespoons almond butter (unsweetened)
- 1 teaspoon pumpkin pie spice
- 1/2 teaspoon vanilla extract
- 10-15 drops liquid stevia (adjust to taste)
- Pinch of salt

1. In a mixing bowl, combine the canned pumpkin puree, melted coconut oil, almond butter, pumpkin pie spice, vanilla extract, liquid stevia, and a pinch of salt. Mix until all ingredients are well combined.

2. Using a silicone mold or an ice cube tray, pour the mixture into individual cavities. You can also use silicone candy molds for fun shapes. Fill each cavity about 3/4 full.

3. Place the mold in the freezer and let the fat bombs set for at least 2 hours, or until they are firm.

4. Once set, remove the fat bombs from the mold and store them in an airtight container in the freezer. Enjoy as needed for a quick, high-fat snack.

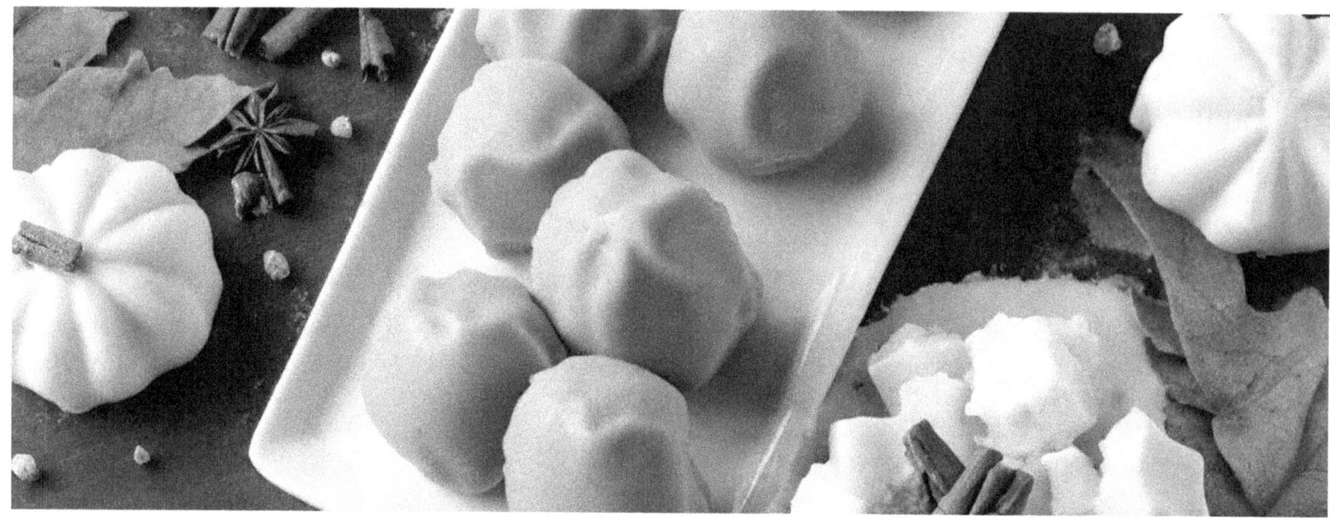

<u>**Tips for Variation:**</u>

- Add a sprinkle of chopped nuts (such as pecans or walnuts) on top of each fat bomb for added crunch and flavor.

- Experiment with different spices like cinnamon, nutmeg, or allspice for a unique twist on the pumpkin spice flavor.

- Consider adding a small amount of unsweetened shredded coconut to the mixture for added texture.

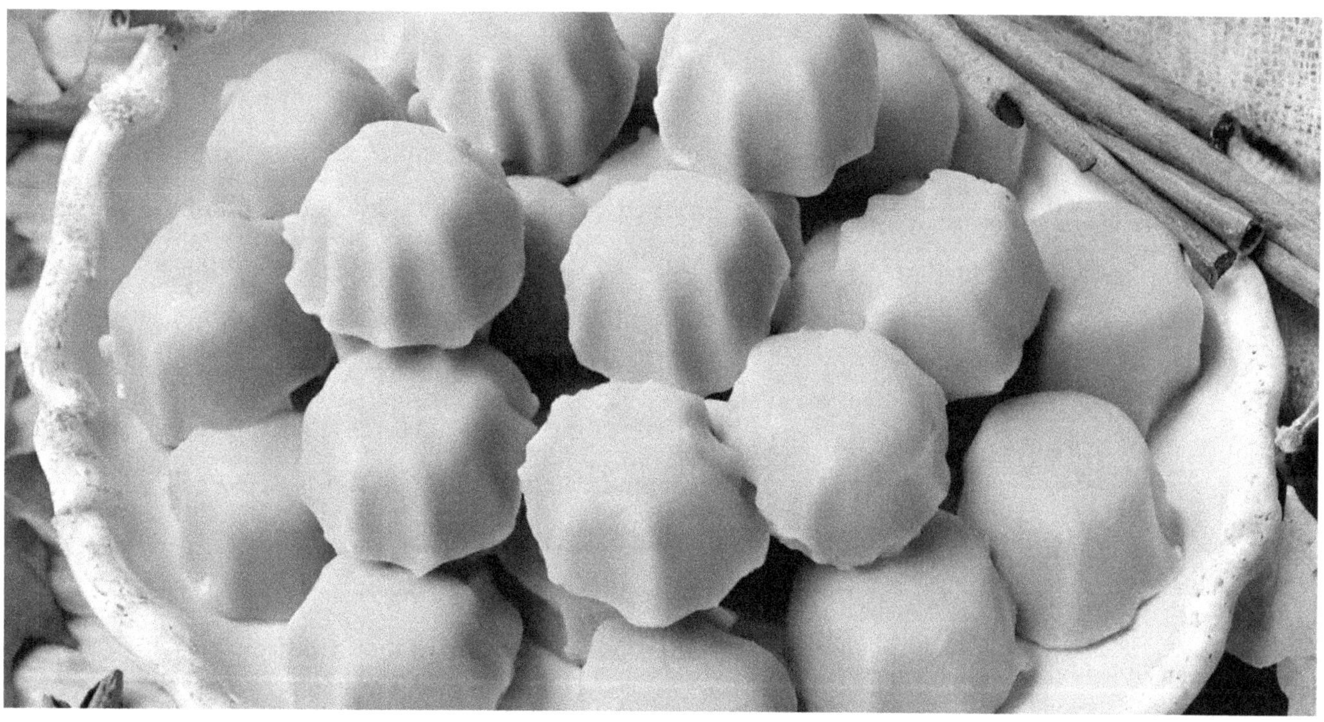

<u>**Nutritional Information:**</u> *Calories: 90 calories, Total Fat: 9g, Saturated Fat: 7g, Cholesterol: 0mg, Sodium: 5mg, Total Carbohydrates: 2g, Dietary Fiber: 1g, Sugars: 1g, Protein: 0.5g*

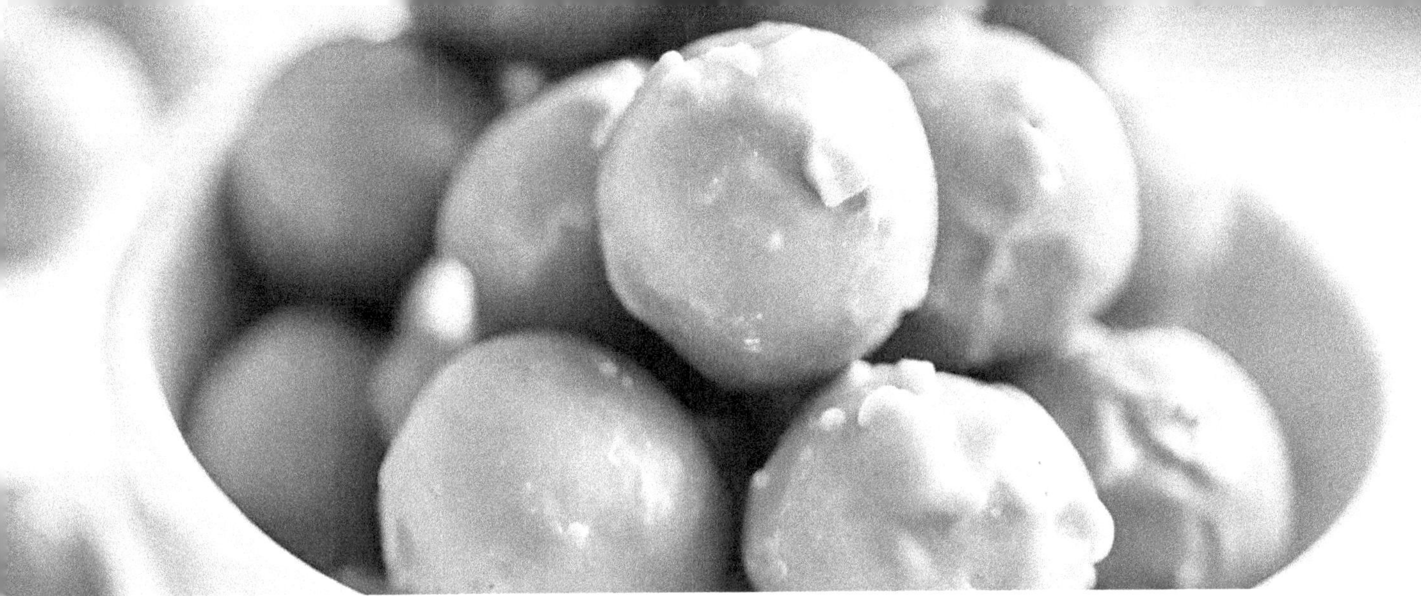

Peanut Butter Protein Balls

SERVINGS: 12   PREP TIME: 15 MINUTES   COOK TIME: 0 MINUTE

- 1/2 cup natural peanut butter (unsweetened)
- 1/4 cup almond flour
- 1/4 cup whey protein powder (unsweetened)
- 2 tablespoons powdered erythritol (or your preferred low-carb sweetener)
- 1/2 teaspoon vanilla extract
- Pinch of salt
- Unsweetened cocoa powder or shredded coconut for coating (optional)

Tips for Variation:

- Use almond butter or another nut or seed butter in place of peanut butter if you have preferences or allergies.
- Add a touch of cinnamon or cocoa powder to the mixture for extra flavor.

1. In a mixing bowl, combine the natural peanut butter, almond flour, whey protein powder, powdered erythritol, vanilla extract, and a pinch of salt. Mix until the ingredients form a dough-like consistency.

2. Take small portions of the mixture and roll them into bite-sized balls. You can make them as big or as small as you prefer.

3. If desired, roll each protein ball in unsweetened cocoa powder or shredded coconut for extra flavor and texture.

4. Place the protein balls on a plate or tray and refrigerate them for at least 30 minutes to firm up.

5. Once chilled, store the Peanut Butter Protein Balls in an airtight container in the refrigerator. Enjoy them as a high-protein snack.

Nutritional Information (per serving): *Calories: 80 calories, Total Fat: 6g, Saturated Fat: 1g, Cholesterol: 0mg, Sodium: 50mg, Total, Carbohydrates: 3g, Dietary Fiber: 1g, Sugars: 1g, Protein: 4g:*

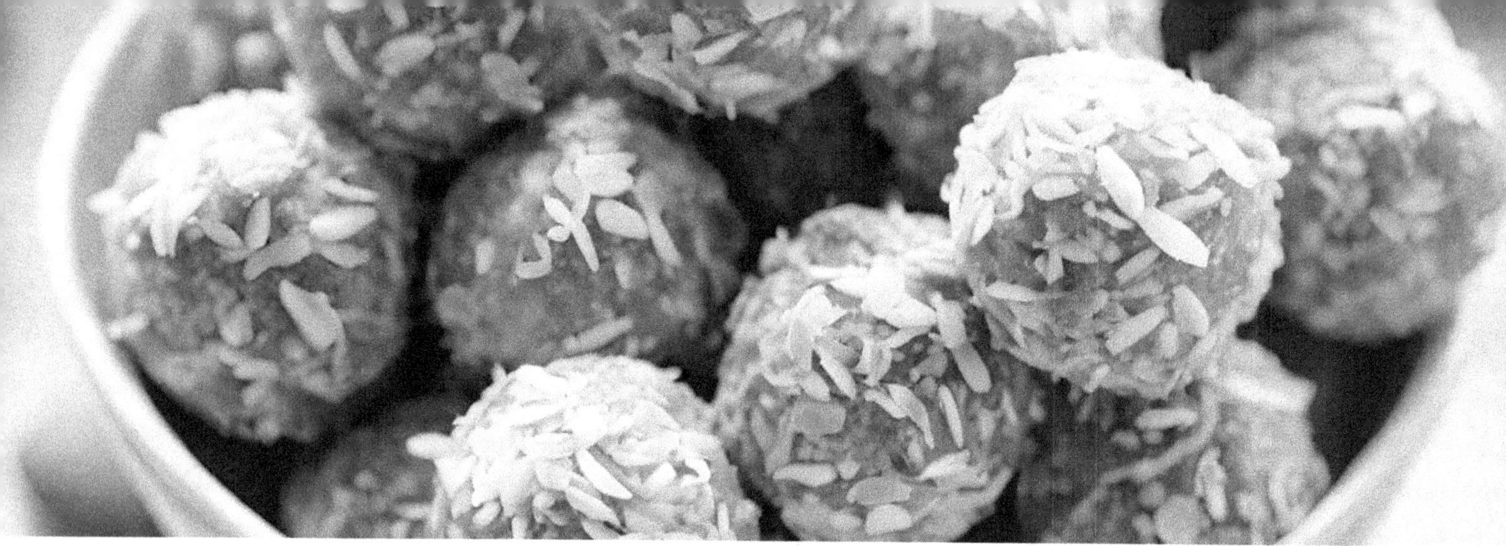

Coconut Almond Energy Balls

SERVINGS: 12   PREP TIME: 15 MINUTES   COOK TIME: 0 MINUTE

INGREDIENTS

- 1/2 cup unsweetened shredded coconut
- 1/4 cup almond flour
- 2 tablespoons coconut oil, melted
- 2 tablespoons powdered erythritol (or your preferred low-carb sweetener)
- 1/2 teaspoon almond extract
- Pinch of salt

Tips for Variation:

- Customize the flavor by adding a few drops of other extracts like vanilla or coconut.
- Incorporate chopped nuts (e.g., almonds, pecans) or unsweetened dark chocolate chips for added texture and taste.
- Adjust the sweetness by adding more or less sweetener to suit your taste.

INSTRUCTIONS

1. In a mixing bowl, combine the unsweetened shredded coconut, almond flour, melted coconut oil, powdered erythritol, almond extract, and a pinch of salt. Mix until the ingredients form a dough-like consistency.

2. Take small portions of the mixture and roll them into bite-sized balls. You can make them as big or as small as you prefer.

3. Place the energy balls on a plate or tray and refrigerate them for at least 30 minutes to firm up.

4. Once chilled, store the Coconut Almond Energy Balls in an airtight container in the refrigerator. Enjoy them as a convenient and satisfying snack.

Nutritional Information (per serving): *Calories: 60 calories, Total Fat: 6g, Saturated Fat: 4g, Cholesterol: 0mg, Sodium: 10mg, Total, Carbohydrates: 2g, Dietary Fiber: 1g, Sugars: 0g, Protein: 1g*

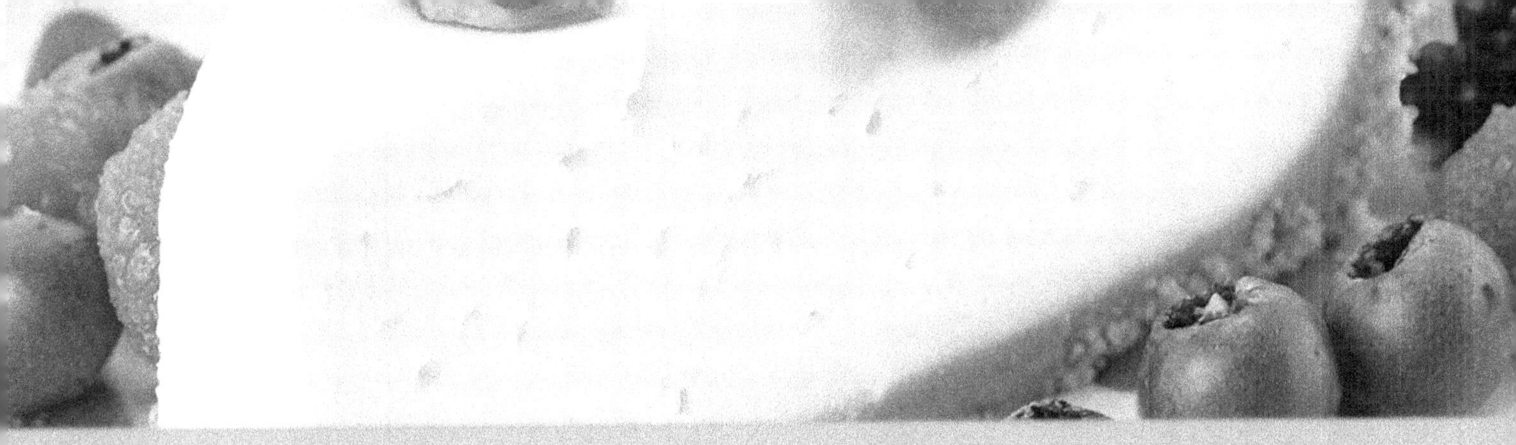

Low-Carb Cheesecake

SERVINGS: 12   PREP TIME: 15 MINUTES   COOK TIME: 40 TO 45 MINUTES

For the Crust:

- 1 cup almond flour
- 2 tablespoons powdered erythritol (or your preferred low-carb sweetener)
- 3 tablespoons unsalted butter, melted

For the Filling:

- 16 ounces (2 packages) cream cheese, softened
- 2/3 cup powdered erythritol (or your preferred low-carb sweetener)
- 2 large eggs
- 1 teaspoon vanilla extract
- Zest of 1 lemon (optional)

For the Crust:

1. Preheat your oven to 325°F (163°C).
2. In a mixing bowl, combine the almond flour, powdered erythritol, and melted butter. Mix until the ingredients form a crumbly mixture.
3. Press the crust mixture into the bottom of an 8-inch (20 cm) spring form pan to create an even layer.

For the Filling:

4. In a separate mixing bowl, beat the softened cream cheese, powdered erythritol, eggs, vanilla extract, and lemon zest (if using) until smooth and well combined.
5. Pour the cream cheese mixture over the crust in the spring form pan, spreading it evenly.
6. Allow the cheesecake to cool at room temperature for about an hour. Then, refrigerate it for at least 4 hours or until it's completely chilled and set.

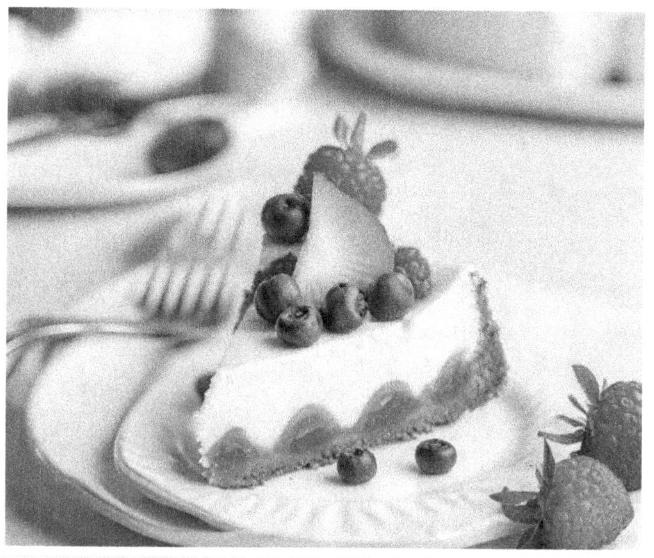

7. Remove the cheesecake from the spring form pan, slice, and serve.

<u>Tips for Variation:</u>

- Top the cheesecake with fresh berries, a sugar-free fruit compote, or a dollop of sugar-free whipped cream for extra flavor and visual appeal.

- Experiment with different extracts (e.g., almond extract or orange extract) to vary the cheesecake's flavor.

- Consider adding a swirl of sugar-free chocolate sauce or caramel sauce for a decadent twist.

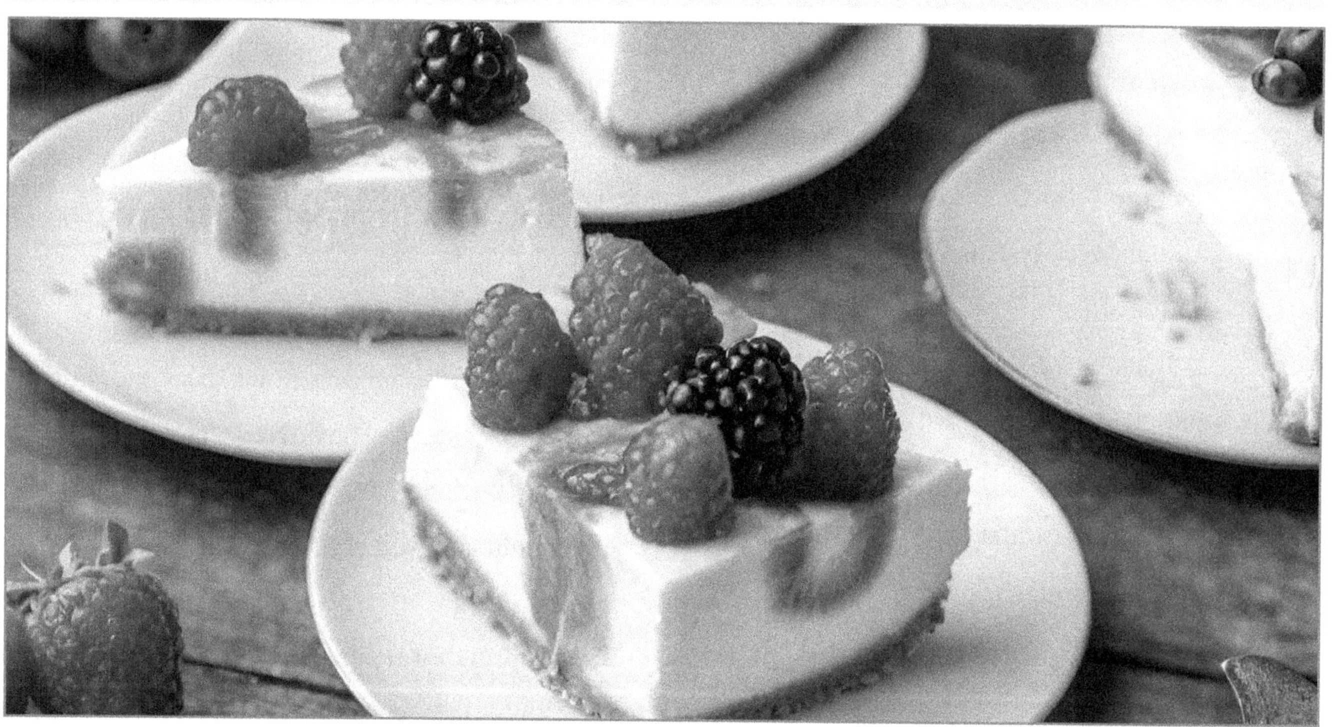

<u>**Nutritional Information:**</u> *Calories: 270 calories, Total Fat: 25g, Saturated Fat: 13g, Cholesterol: 90mg, Sodium: 170mg, Total Carbohydrates: 4g, Dietary Fiber: 1g, Sugars: 1g, Protein: 6g*

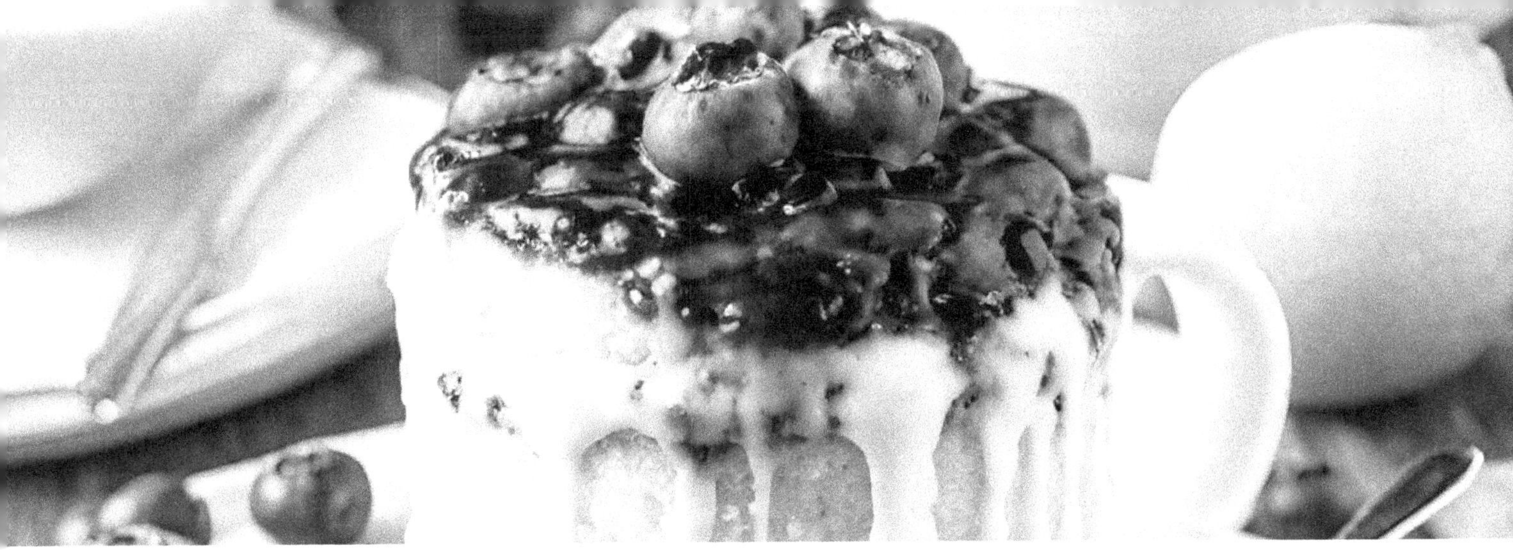

Lemon Blueberry Mug Cake

- 2 tablespoons almond flour
- 1 tablespoon coconut flour
- 1 tablespoon powdered erythritol (or your preferred low-carb sweetener)
- 1/4 teaspoon baking powder
- Pinch of salt
- Zest of 1 lemon
- 1 large egg
- 2 tablespoons unsalted butter, melted
- 1 tablespoon lemon juice
- 1/4 cup fresh or frozen blueberries

1. In a microwave-safe mug, combine the almond flour, coconut flour, powdered erythritol, baking powder, pinch of salt, and lemon zest. Mix well.
2. Add the egg, melted butter, and lemon juice to the dry ingredients. Mix until the batter is well combined.
3. Gently fold in the blueberries into the batter.
4. Microwave the mug on high for 1-2 minutes, or until the cake has risen and is set in the center. Cooking time may vary depending on your microwave's wattage.
5. Let the mug cake cool for a minute or two before enjoying.

Tips for Variation:

- Swap out the blueberries for other low-carb berries like raspberries or blackberries.
- Add a small dollop of sugar-free whipped cream or a drizzle of lemon glaze made from lemon juice and powdered erythritol for extra flavor.

Nutritional Information (per serving): *Calories: 330 calories, Total Fat: 29g, Saturated Fat: 14g, Cholesterol: 200mg, Sodium: 380mg, Total Carbohydrates: 10g, Dietary Fiber: 4g, Sugars: 3g, Protein:*

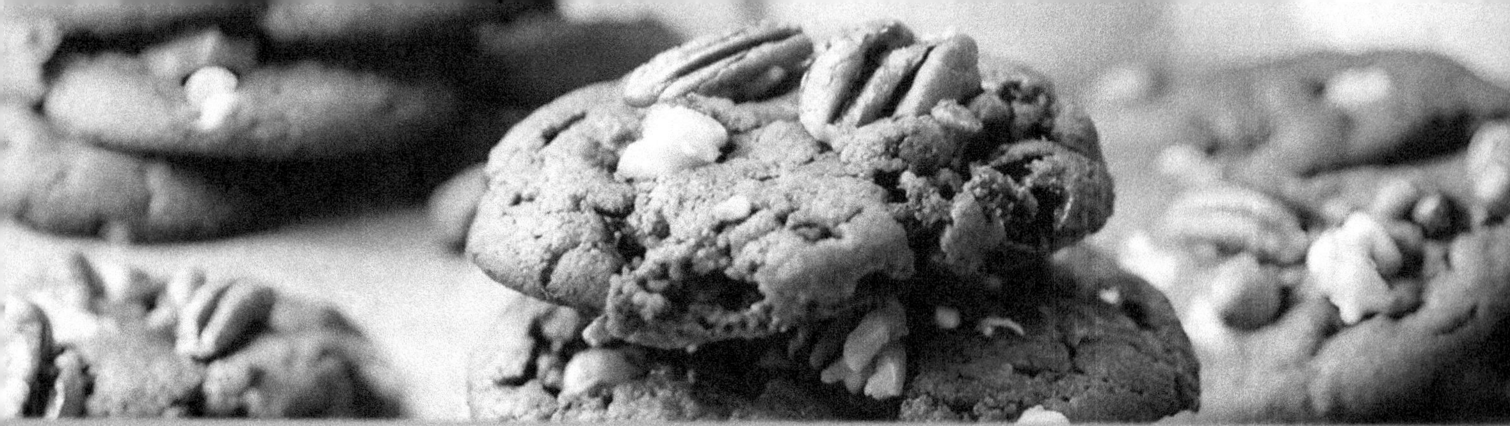

Chocolate Pecan Cookies

SERVINGS: 12   PREP TIME: 15 MINUTES   COOK TIME: 10 TO 12 MINUTES

INGREDIENTS

- 1 cup almond flour
- 1/4 cup unsweetened cocoa powder
- 1/4 cup powdered erythritol (or your preferred low-carb sweetener)
- 1/4 teaspoon baking soda
- Pinch of salt
- 1/4 cup unsalted butter, softened
- 1/2 teaspoon vanilla extract
- 1 large egg
- 1/4 cup chopped pecans
- 2 tablespoons sugar-free chocolate chips (optional)

INSTRUCTIONS

1. Preheat your oven to 350°F (175°C) and line a baking sheet with parchment paper.

2. In a mixing bowl, whisk together the almond flour, unsweetened cocoa powder, powdered erythritol, baking soda, and a pinch of salt.

3. In a separate bowl, cream together the softened unsalted butter and vanilla extract. Add the egg and continue to mix until well combined.

4. Gradually add the dry ingredient mixture to the wet ingredients, mixing until a cookie dough forms.

5. Gently fold in the chopped pecans and sugar-free chocolate chips (if using) into the cookie dough.

6. Using a tablespoon, scoop portions of dough onto the prepared baking sheet, spacing them apart.

7. Flatten each cookie slightly with the back of a fork or the palm of your hand.

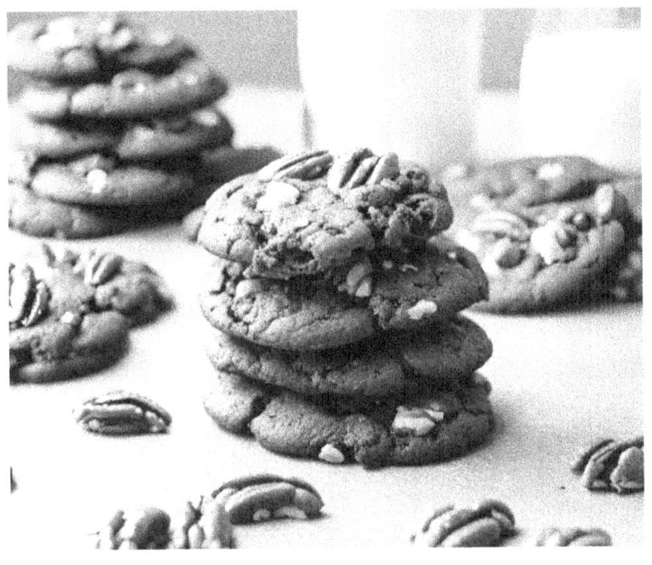

8. Bake in the preheated oven for 10-12 minutes or until the edges are firm and the cookies have set.

9. Allow the cookies to cool on the baking sheet for a few minutes before transferring them to a wire rack to cool completely.

Tips for Variation:

- Add chopped walnuts or almonds for extra nutty flavor and crunch.

- For a different twist, mix in unsweetened shredded coconut or orange zest.

- Experiment with different low-carb sweeteners like stevia or monk fruit sweetener to suit your taste.

- If you prefer a softer cookie, reduce the baking time slightly.

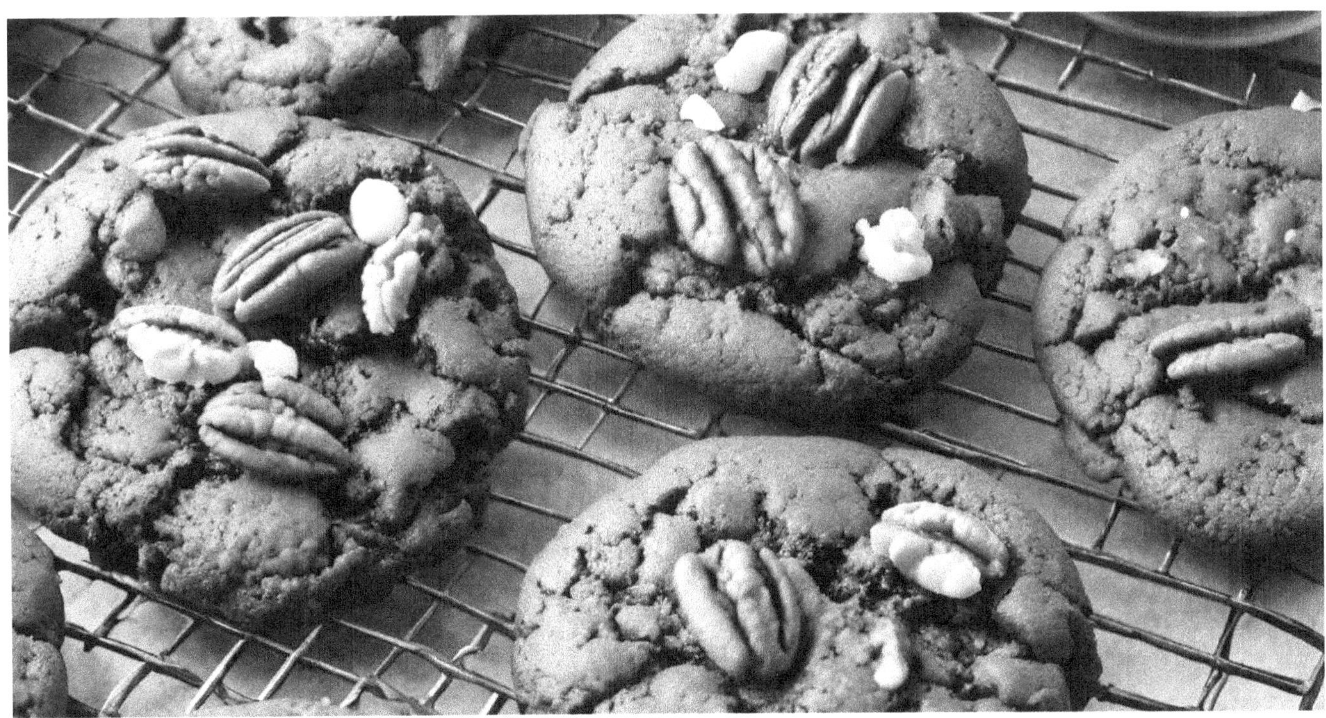

Nutritional Information: *Calories: 100 calories, Total Fat: 9g, Saturated Fat: 3g, Cholesterol: 20mg, Sodium: 50mg, Total Carbohydrates: 4g, Dietary Fiber: 2g, Sugars: 1g, Protein: 2g*

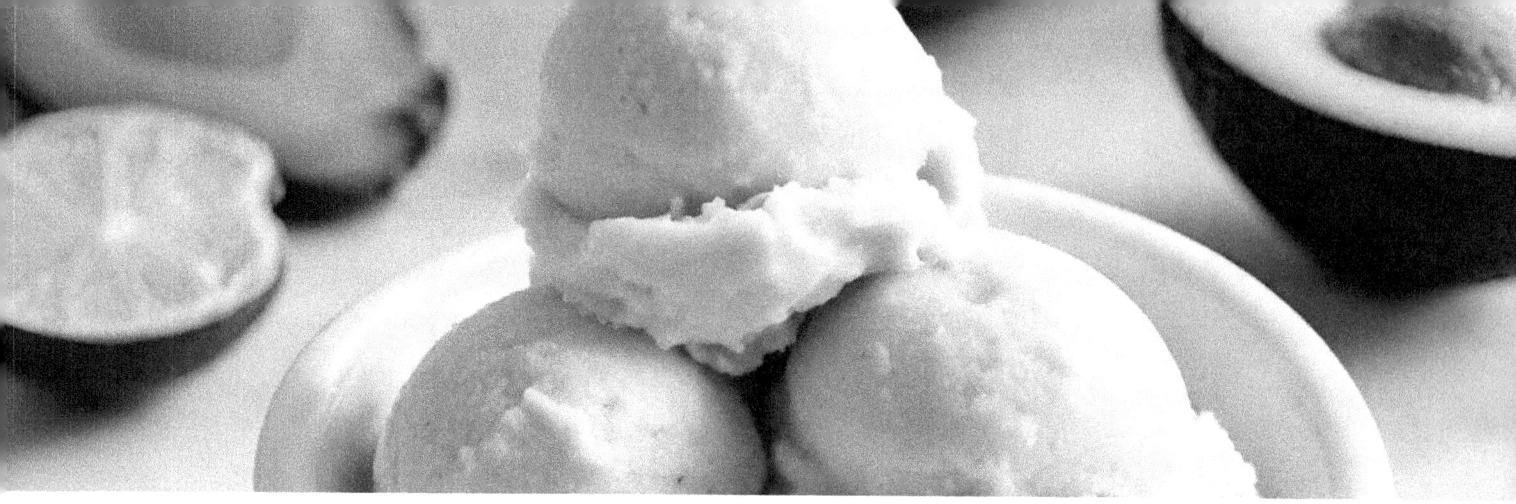

Avocado Lime Sorbet

INGREDIENTS

- 2 ripe avocados, peeled and pitted
- 1/4 cup fresh lime juice (approximately 2-3 limes)
- Zest of 1 lime
- 1/4 cup powdered erythritol (or your preferred low-carb sweetener)
- 1/4 cup unsweetened almond milk (or coconut milk)
- 1/2 teaspoon vanilla extract
- Pinch of salt

Tips for Variation:

- Add a touch of mint extract or fresh mint leaves for a refreshing twist on the flavor.
- Create a tropical variation by blending in unsweetened shredded coconut or pineapple chunks.

INSTRUCTIONS

1. In a blender or food processor, combine the peeled avocados, fresh lime juice, lime zest, powdered erythritol, unsweetened almond milk, vanilla extract, and a pinch of salt.

2. Blend the mixture until it becomes a smooth, creamy sorbet base. You may need to scrape down the sides of the blender to ensure everything is well mixed.

3. Taste the sorbet base and adjust the sweetness if needed by adding more sweetener.

4. Pour the sorbet base into a freezer-safe container and cover it. Place it in the freezer for at least 4 hours or until it's firm.

5. When ready to serve, scoop the sorbet into bowls or cones. Garnish with lime zest or fresh lime slices if desired.

Nutritional Information (per serving): Calories: 160 calories, Total Fat: 14g, Saturated Fat: 2g, Cholesterol: 0mg, Sodium: 50mg, Total Carbohydrates: 10g, Dietary Fiber: 7g, Sugars: 1g, Protein: 2g

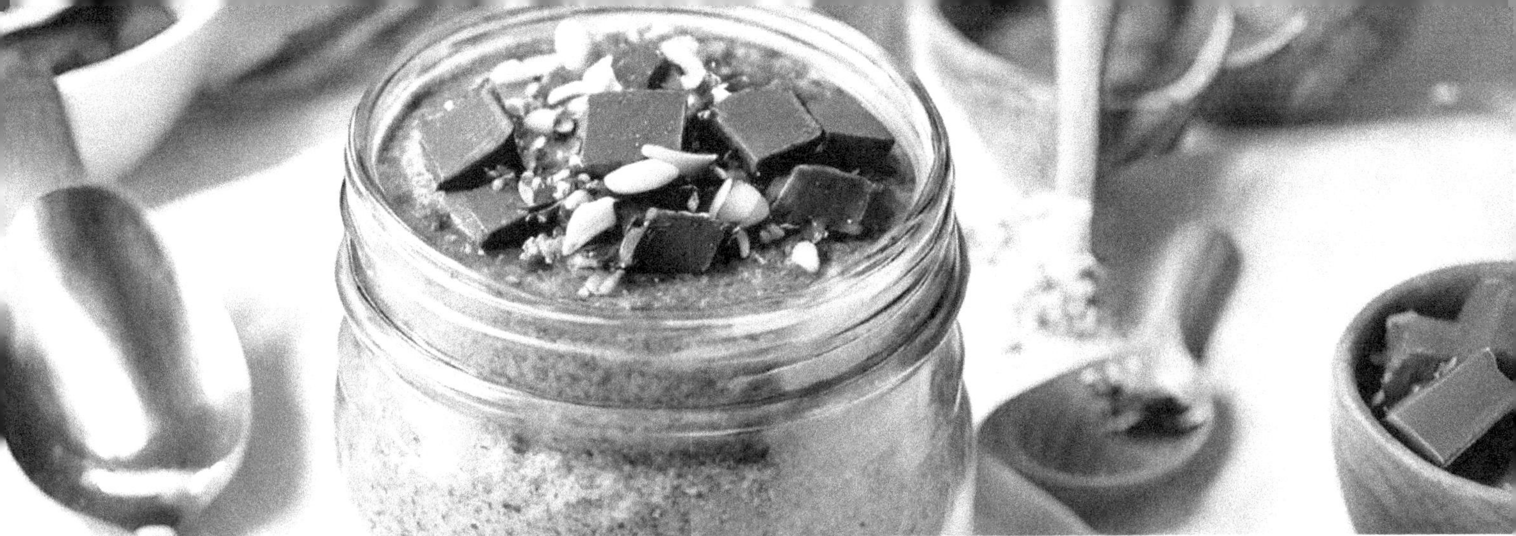

Coconut Chocolate Chia Pudding

- 1/4 cup chia seeds
- 1 cup unsweetened coconut milk (canned or from a carton)
- 2 tablespoons unsweetened cocoa powder
- 2-3 tablespoons powdered erythritol (or your preferred low-carb sweetener)
- 1/2 teaspoon vanilla extract
- A pinch of salt
- Unsweetened shredded coconut and dark chocolate shavings for garnish (optional)

1. In a mixing bowl, combine the chia seeds, unsweetened cocoa powder, powdered erythritol, and a pinch of salt. Mix them together to evenly distribute the cocoa powder and sweetener.

2. Pour in the unsweetened coconut milk and vanilla extract into the dry mixture. Stir well to ensure that the chia seeds are fully immersed in the liquid.

3. Taste the mixture and adjust the sweetness by adding more powdered erythritol if desired. Remember that the sweetness may slightly mellow as the pudding sets.

4. Cover the bowl with plastic wrap or transfer the mixture to individual serving containers. Place the pudding in the refrigerator for at least 2-3 hours or overnight. Stir it once after about 30 minutes to prevent clumping.

5. When ready to serve, garnish the pudding with unsweetened shredded coconut and dark chocolate shavings if desired.

<u>**Tips for Variation:**</u>

- Add fresh berries (e.g., strawberries, raspberries) or sliced almonds for added flavor and texture. Be mindful of the carb content if you choose to add fruit.

- Stir in chopped nuts like almonds, pecans, or walnuts for a delightful crunch.

- Experiment with a dash of cinnamon or a pinch of chili powder for a unique twist on the flavor.

- Enhance the coconut flavor by adding a few drops of coconut extract or a sprinkle of unsweetened shredded coconut to the pudding mixture before refrigerating.

- You can add a scoop of unflavored or chocolate-flavored whey protein powder for added protein content.

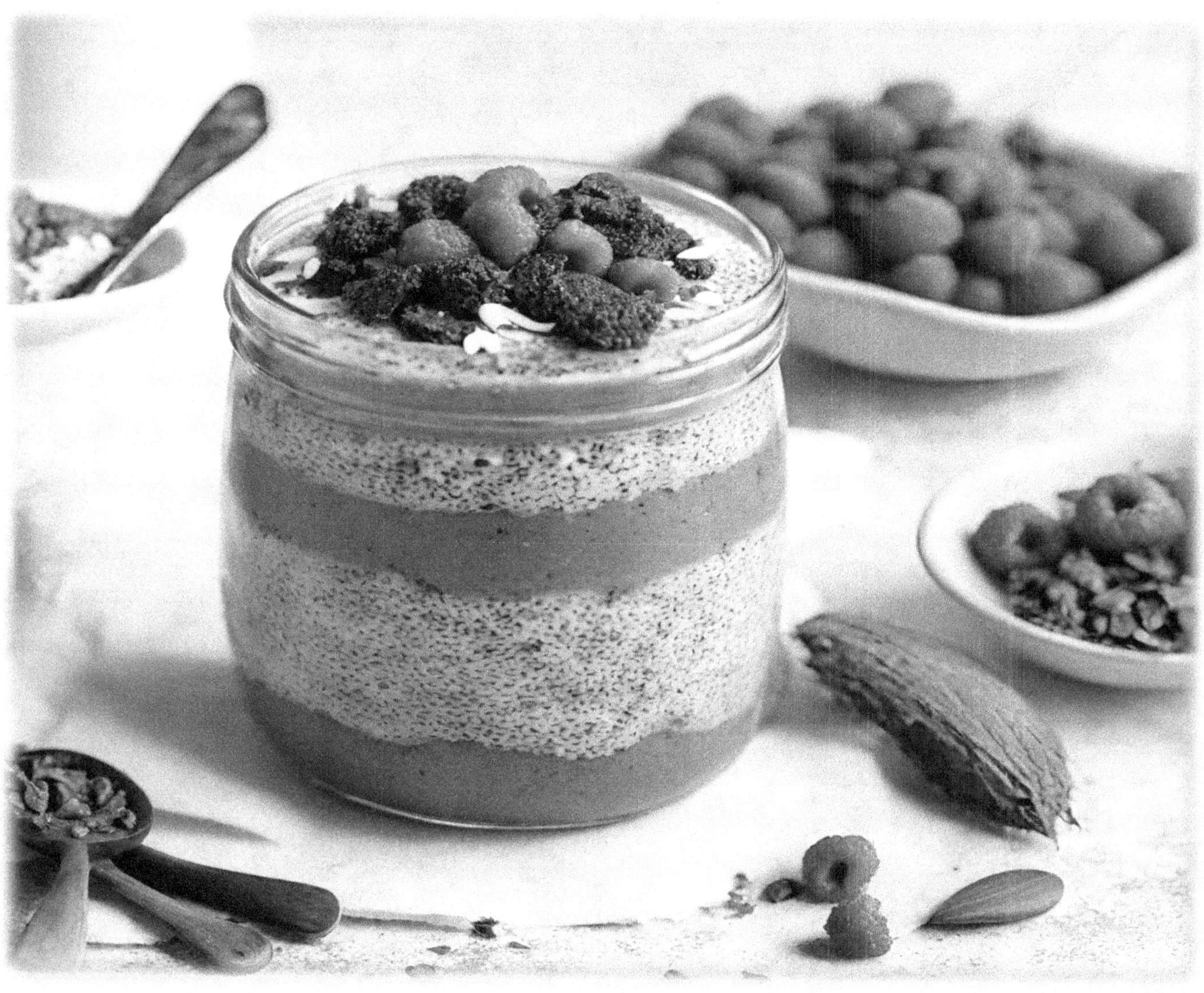

<u>**Nutritional Information:**</u> *Calories: 180 calories, Total Fat: 14g, Saturated Fat: 7g, Cholesterol: 0mg, Sodium: 70mg, Total Carbohydrates: 12g, Dietary Fiber: 9g, Sugars: 1g, Protein: 4g*

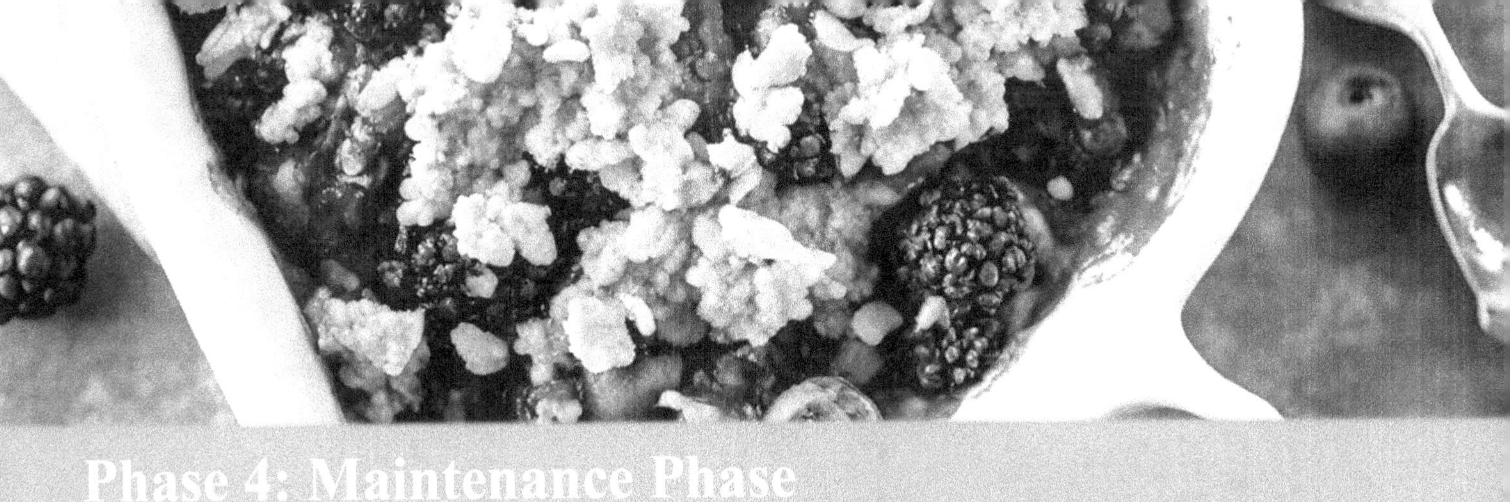

Low-Carb Berry Crisp

SERVINGS: 4   PREP TIME: 10 MINUTES   COOK TIME: 25 TO 30 MINUTES

For the Berry Filling:

- 2 cups mixed berries (e.g., strawberries, blueberries, raspberries)
- 2 tablespoons powdered erythritol (or your preferred low-carb sweetener)
- 1 tablespoon lemon juice
- 1/2 teaspoon vanilla extract

For the Crisp Topping:

- 1/2 cup almond flour
- 1/4 cup unsweetened shredded coconut
- 2 tablespoons powdered erythritol (or your preferred low-carb sweetener)
- 2 tablespoons cold unsalted butter, cubed
- 1/4 teaspoon cinnamon
- Pinch of salt

For the Berry Filling:

1. Preheat your oven to 350°F (175°C).
2. In a mixing bowl, combine the mixed berries, powdered erythritol, lemon juice, and vanilla extract. Toss to coat the berries evenly.
3. Place the berry mixture in a baking dish (e.g., 8x8 inches) and spread it out evenly.

For the Crisp Topping:

4. In a separate mixing bowl, combine the almond flour, shredded coconut, powdered erythritol, cubed cold butter, cinnamon, and a pinch of salt. Use your fingers or a pastry cutter to blend the ingredients together until they resemble coarse crumbs.
5. Sprinkle the crisp topping evenly over the berry mixture in the baking dish.
6. Bake in the preheated oven for 25-30 minutes or until the topping is golden brown and the berry filling is bubbly.

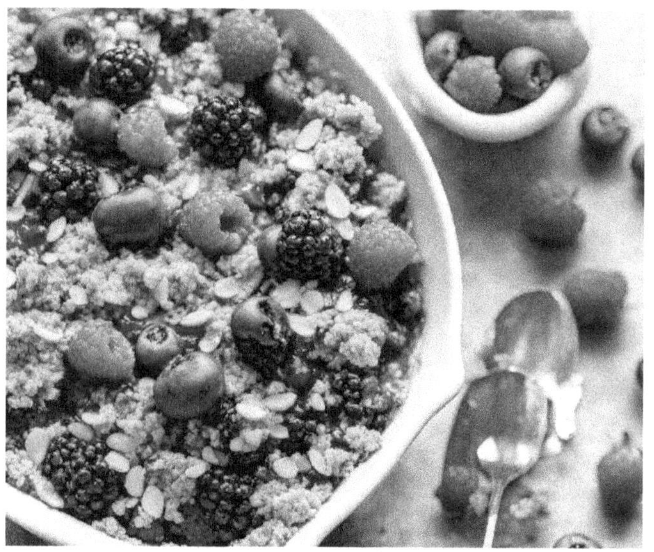

7. Allow the berry crisp to cool for a few minutes before serving.

<u>Tips for Variation:</u>

- Add a scoop of sugar-free vanilla ice cream or a dollop of unsweetened whipped cream when serving for extra indulgence.

- Experiment with different combinations of berries based on your preferences and seasonal availability.

- Include chopped nuts like almonds or pecans in the crisp topping for added crunch and flavor.

- If you prefer a sweeter filling, adjust the amount of sweetener to taste.

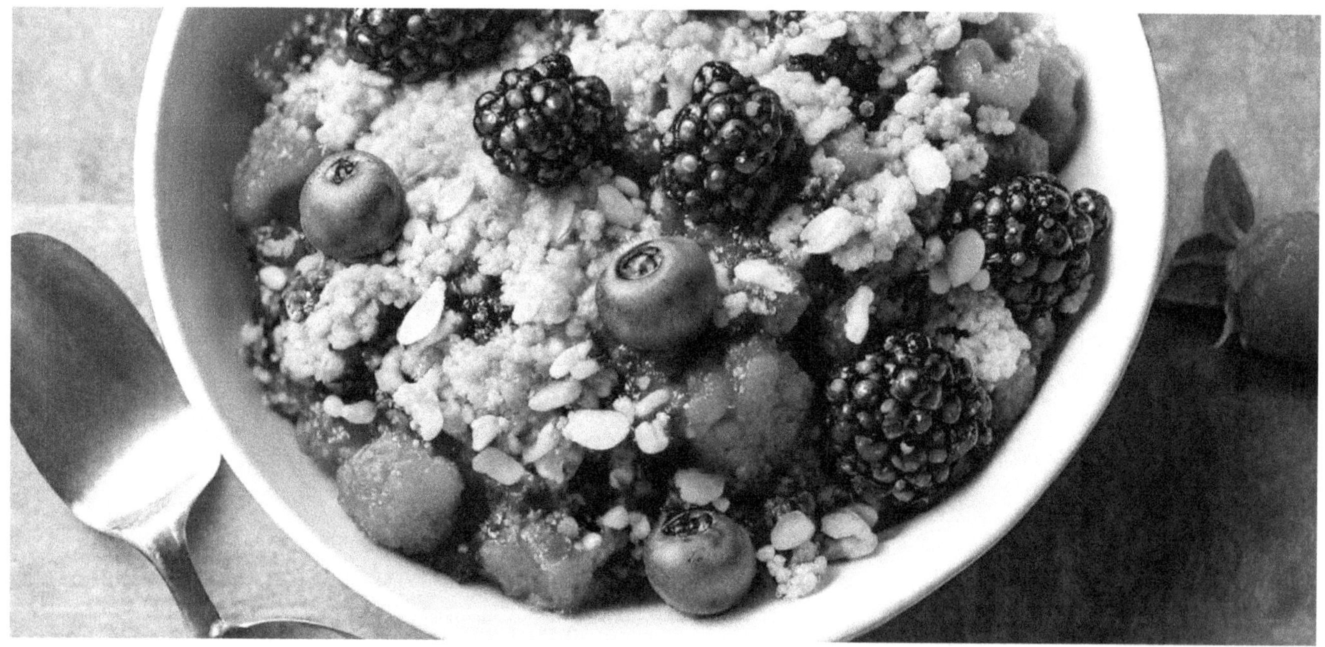

<u>**Nutritional Information:**</u> *Calories: 180 calories, Total Fat: 15g, Saturated Fat: 6g, Cholesterol: 15mg, Sodium: 50mg, Total Carbohydrates: 10g, Dietary Fiber: 4g, Sugars: 4g, Protein: 3g*

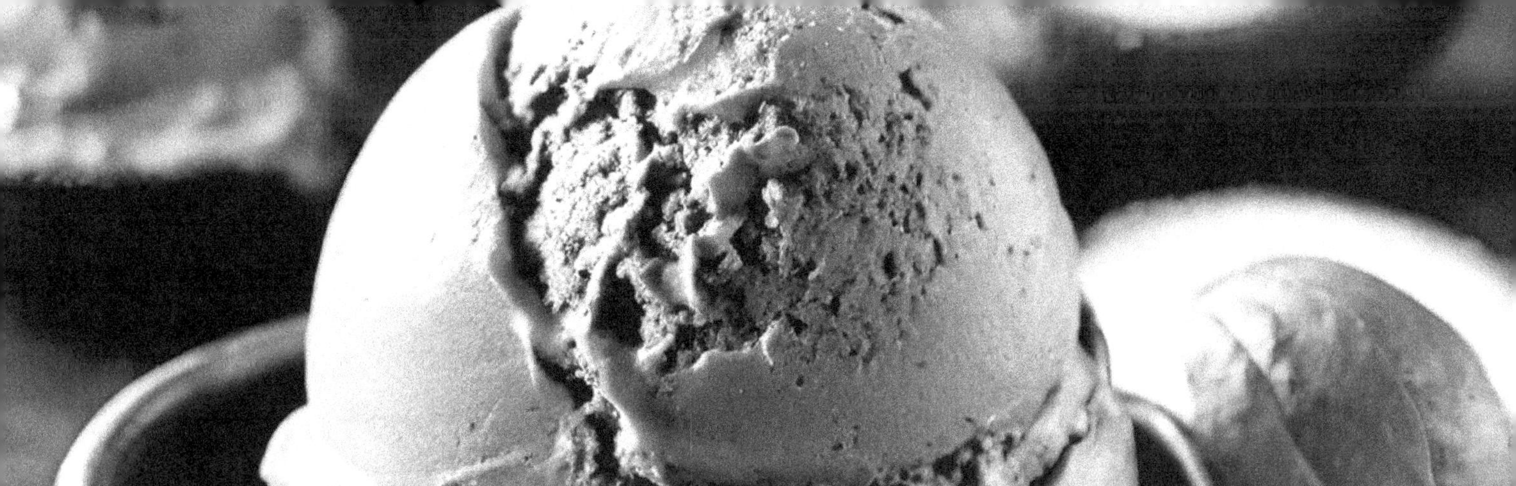

Chocolate Avocado Ice Cream

SERVINGS: 4   PREP TIME: 10 MINUTES   COOK TIME: 4 HOURS

- 2 ripe avocados, peeled and pitted
- 1/2 cup unsweetened cocoa powder
- 1/2 cup powdered erythritol (or your preferred low-carb sweetener)
- 1 cup unsweetened almond milk (or coconut milk)
- 1 teaspoon vanilla extract
- Pinch of salt
- 1/4 cup sugar-free chocolate chips (optional)

1. In a blender or food processor, combine the peeled avocados, unsweetened cocoa powder, powdered erythritol, unsweetened almond milk, vanilla extract, and a pinch of salt. Blend until the mixture is smooth and creamy.
2. Taste the ice cream mixture and adjust the sweetness by adding more powdered erythritol if needed.
3. If desired, fold in sugar-free chocolate chips into the ice cream mixture for added chocolatey goodness.
4. Pour the ice cream mixture into a freezer-safe container and cover it. Place it in the freezer for at least 4 hours or until it's firm.
5. When ready to serve, scoop the Chocolate Avocado Ice Cream into bowls or cones.

Tips for Variation:

- Customize the ice cream by adding your favorite low-carb mix-ins, such as chopped nuts, unsweetened shredded coconut, or a swirl of sugar-free caramel sauce.

Nutritional Information (per serving): Calories: 200 calories, Total Fat: 15g, Saturated Fat: 4g, Cholesterol: 0mg, Sodium: 60mg, Total Carbohydrates: 16g, Dietary Fiber: 9g, Sugars: 1g, Protein: 4g

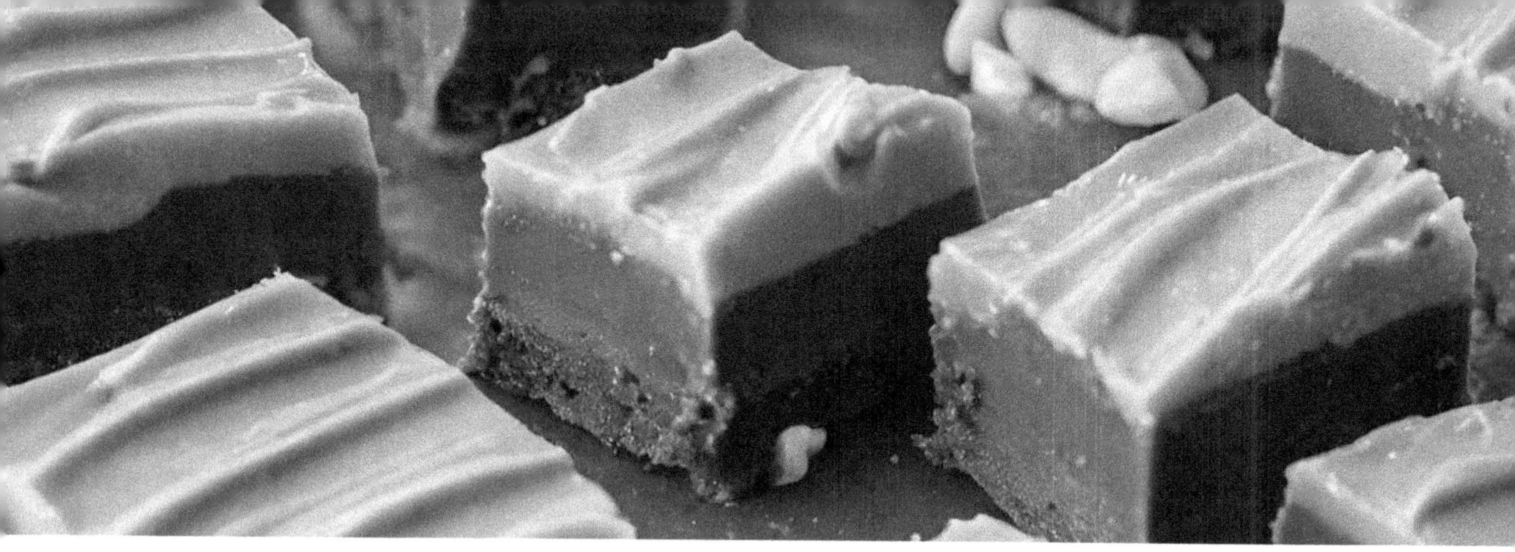

Peanut Butter Chocolate Fudge

SERVINGS: 12   PREP TIME: 10 MINUTES   COOK TIME: 2 TO 3 MINUTES

INGREDIENTS

- 1/2 cup natural peanut butter (unsweetened)
- 1/4 cup coconut oil, melted
- 1/4 cup unsweetened cocoa powder
- 1/4 cup powdered erythritol (or your preferred low-carb sweetener)
- 1/2 teaspoon vanilla extract
- Pinch of salt
- Chopped peanuts or sugar-free chocolate chips for garnish (optional)

Tips for Variation:

- Drizzle melted sugar-free dark chocolate on top of the fudge for an extra layer of chocolate flavor.
- Add a dash of cinnamon or a pinch of sea salt to enhance the taste.

INSTRUCTIONS

1. Line a small container or dish (such as an 8x4-inch loaf pan) with parchment paper, leaving some overhang for easy removal.
2. In a mixing bowl, combine the natural peanut butter, melted coconut oil, unsweetened cocoa powder, powdered erythritol, vanilla extract, and a pinch of salt. Stir until all the ingredients are well combined.
3. Pour the peanut butter chocolate mixture into the prepared mold, spreading it out evenly.
4. If desired, sprinkle chopped peanuts or sugar-free chocolate chips on top of the fudge.
5. Place the mold in the refrigerator and let the fudge set for at least 2-3 hours or until it's firm.
6. Once set, use the parchment paper overhang to lift the fudge out of the container. Cut it into small squares or bars.

Nutritional Information (per serving): *Calories: 120 calories, Total Fat: 11g, Saturated Fat: 5g, Cholesterol: 0mg, Sodium: 50mg, Total Carbohydrates: 4g, Dietary Fiber: 2g, Sugars: 0g, Protein: 3g*

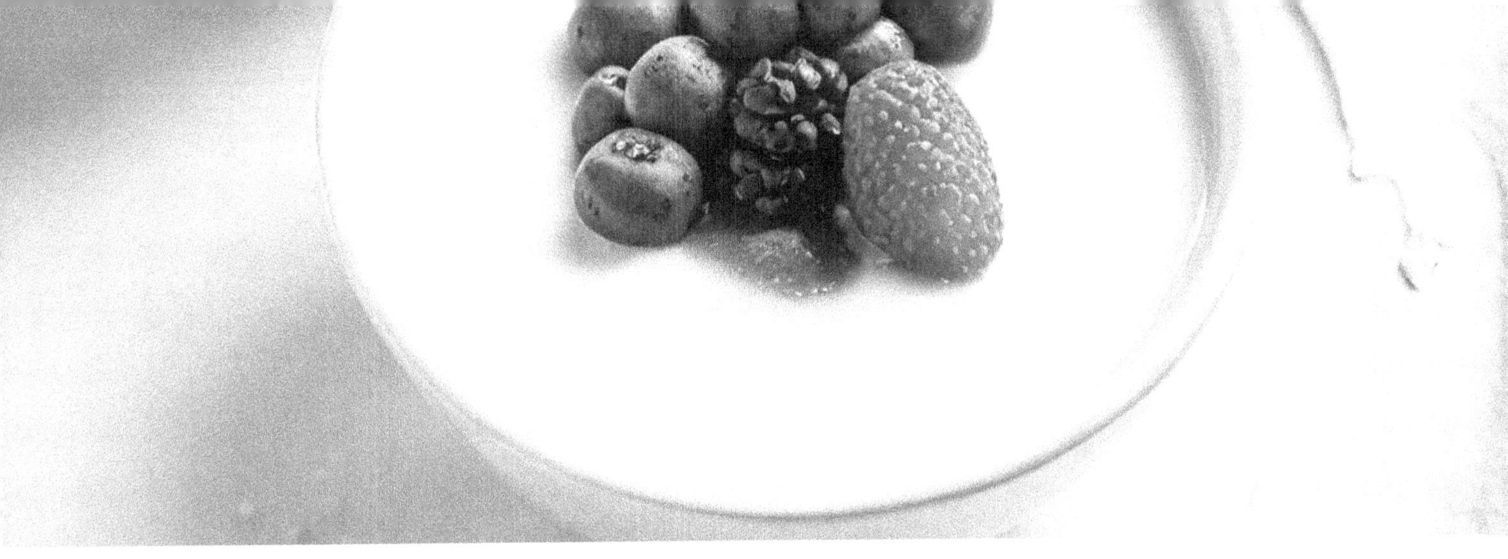

Vanilla Almond Panna Cotta

SERVINGS: 4   PREP TIME: 10 MINUTES   COOK TIME 4 HOURS

- 1 cup unsweetened almond milk
- 1/2 cup heavy cream
- 1/4 cup powdered erythritol (or your preferred low-carb sweetener)
- 1 teaspoon vanilla extract
- 1 packet unflavored gelatin (about 2.5 teaspoons)
- 2 tablespoons cold water
- Sliced almonds and a drizzle of sugar-free caramel sauce for garnish (optional)

Tips for Variation:

- Infuse the panna cotta with additional flavors by steeping a herbal tea bag (e.g., chamomile or lavender) in the almond milk mixture before heating.

1. In a small bowl, sprinkle the unflavored gelatin over 2 tablespoons of cold water. Let it sit for 5 minutes to bloom.
2. In a saucepan, combine the unsweetened almond milk, heavy cream, powdered erythritol, and vanilla extract. Heat the mixture over low-medium heat until it's warm but not boiling, stirring to dissolve the sweetener.
3. Once the gelatin has bloomed, microwave it for about 10 seconds or until it becomes a liquid. Stir the liquid gelatin into the warm almond milk mixture until fully dissolved.
4. Remove the mixture from the heat and pour it into individual ramekins or molds.
5. Refrigerate the panna cotta for at least 4 hours or until it's set and firm.
6. When ready to serve, garnish with sliced almonds and a drizzle of sugar-free caramel sauce if desired.

Nutritional Information (per serving): Calories: 250 calories, Total Fat: 23g, Saturated Fat: 13g, Cholesterol: 80mg, Sodium: 15mg, Total Carbohydrates: 4g, Dietary Fiber: 1g, Sugars: 0g, Protein: 5g

Notes:

Your
Observation:

Progress
Report:

Chapter Eight: Four-Week Meal Plan

Day	Breakfast	Lunch	Dinner	Snack
		WEEK 1		
1	Keto Sausage Egg Cups	Three-Style Chicken Breast	Grilled Lemon Herb Chicken	Peanut Butter Protein Balls
2	Egg Casserole	Avocado Egg Salad	Baked Salmon with Dill Sauce	Coconut Almond Energy Balls
3	Vegan Keto Coconut Protein Shake	Grilled Pork Belly	Sautéed Shrimp with Garlic and Spinach	Greek Yogurt Parfait
4	Keto Turkey Breakfast Meatloaf Parfait	Keto Turkey Meatloaf	Turkey and Avocado Lettuce Wraps	Buffalo Cauliflower Bites
5	Keto Bacon Egg Muffins	Beef Tenderloin & Vegetable Stir Fry	Zucchini Noodles with Pesto and Grilled Chicken	Stuffed Mushrooms
6	Chocolate & Strawberry Smoothie	Spicy Tofu Steak	Cauliflower Crust Pizza	Cheese and Pepperoni
7	Scrambled Eggs with Bacon, Green Bell Peppers and Tomato	Bacon-Egg Salad Flatout Wrap	Grilled Steak with Asparagus	Almond Butter and Celery
		WEEK 2		
8	Berry Parfait	Loaded Broccoli Salad	Stuffed Bell Peppers	Sliced Veggies with Ranch Dressing
9	Fennel, Carrot and Turkey Hash	Salmon-Stuffed Avocados	Cabbage Rolls with Ground Beef	Protein Smoothie
10	Chocolate Protein Pancakes	Arugula, Chicken & Melon Salad with Sumac Dressing	Stir-Fried Tofu with Vegetables	Cottage Cheese with Berries
11	Pepperoni Pizza Frittata	Tuna Salad with Egg	Grilled Pork Chops with Roasted Brussels Sprouts	Bacon-Wrapped Avocado
12	Leek Quiche	Garlic Ranch Dip with Sumac Dressing	Grilled Lamb Chops with Mint Sauce	Cucumber Bites

13	Spinach and Mushroom Omelette	Spinach & Artichoke-Stuffed Portobello Mushrooms	Baked Cod with Lemon Butter Sauce	Deviled Eggs
14	Avocado and Bacon Scramble	Chopped Power Salad with Chicken	Spaghetti Squash with Meatballs	Zucchini Chips

WEEK 3

15	Keto Sausage Egg Cups	Three-Style Chicken Breast	Grilled Lemon Herb Chicken	Peanut Butter Protein Balls
16	Egg Casserole	Avocado Egg Salad	Baked Salmon with Dill Sauce	Coconut Almond Energy Balls
17	Vegan Keto Coconut Protein Shake	Grilled Pork Belly	Sautéed Shrimp with Garlic and Spinach	Greek Yogurt Parfait
18	Keto Turkey Breakfast Meatloaf Parfait	Keto Turkey Meatloaf	Turkey and Avocado Lettuce Wraps	Buffalo Cauliflower Bites
19	Keto Bacon Egg Muffins	Beef Tenderloin & Vegetable Stir Fry	Zucchini Noodles with Pesto and Grilled Chicken	Stuffed Mushrooms
20	Chocolate & Strawberry Smoothie	Spicy Tofu Steak	Cauliflower Crust Pizza	Cheese and Pepperoni
21	Scrambled Eggs with Bacon, Green Bell Peppers and Tomato	Bacon-Egg Salad Flatout Wrap	Grilled Steak with Asparagus	Almond Butter and Celery

WEEK 4

22	Berry Parfait	Loaded Broccoli Salad	Stuffed Bell Peppers	Sliced Veggies with Ranch Dressing
23	Fennel, Carrot and Turkey Hash	Salmon-Stuffed Avocados	Cabbage Rolls with Ground Beef	Protein Smoothie
24	Chocolate Protein Pancakes	Arugula, Chicken & Melon Salad with Sumac Dressing	Stir-Fried Tofu with Vegetables	Cottage Cheese with Berries
25	Pepperoni Pizza Frittata	Tuna Salad with Egg	Grilled Pork Chops with Roasted Brussels Sprouts	Bacon-Wrapped Avocado
26	Leek Quiche	Garlic Ranch Dip with Sumac Dressing	Grilled Lamb Chops with Mint Sauce	Cucumber Bites

| 27 | Spinach and Mushroom Omelette | Spinach & Artichoke-Stuffed Portobello Mushrooms | Baked Cod with Lemon Butter Sauce | Deviled Eggs |
| 28 | Avocado and Bacon Scramble | Chopped Power Salad with Chicken | Spaghetti Squash with Meatballs | Zucchini Chips |

Feel free to adjust the meal plan according to your preferences and dietary needs. Enjoy your meals!

Grocery Shopping List

Embarking on a new dietary journey, whether it's for health reasons or a desire to explore new culinary horizons, often begins with a well-stocked pantry and fridge. As you dive into the world of Atkins Diet recipes, ensuring you have the right ingredients on hand is key to success. From lean proteins to vibrant vegetables and flavorful spices, this comprehensive grocery shopping list will equip you with everything you need to create delicious and satisfying meals while following the Atkins Diet.

1. Proteins

- Sausage (for Keto Sausage Egg Cups)
- Eggs
- Turkey sausage (for Keto Turkey Breakfast Meatloaf Parfait)
- Bacon
- Chicken breasts
- Pork belly
- Ground turkey
- Shrimp
- Steak (such as tenderloin or flank)
- Lamb chops
- Salmon fillets
- Cod fillets
- Ground beef
- Tofu

2. Dairy and Alternatives

- Coconut milk (for Vegan Keto Coconut Protein Shake)
- Heavy cream
- Greek yogurt
- Cheddar cheese
- Provolone cheese
- Gruyere cheese
- Cream cheese
- Cottage cheese
- Almond milk
- Butter
- Parmesan cheese

3. Vegetables

- Snow peas
- Broccoli

	– Red bell pepper – Spinach – Mushrooms – Zucchini – Cauliflower – Asparagus – Bell peppers (various colors) – Avocado – Leeks – Carrots – Scallions or spring onions – Brussels sprouts – Portobello mushrooms – Arugula – Melon – Cucumber – Garlic – Tomatoes
4. Fruits	– Strawberries – Raspberries – Lemons – Berries (for snacking and parfaits)
5. Herbs and Spices:	– Vanilla extract – Cilantro – Basil – Parsley – Dill – Sumac – Ginger – Cumin – Cayenne pepper – Paprika
6. Pantry Staples	– Sucralose-based sweetener (sugar substitute) – Cornstarch – Low-sodium soy sauce – Hoisin sauce or oyster sauce – Shaoxing cooking wine – Pure sesame oil – Light brown sugar – Lemon juice – Black pepper – Garlic powder – Ranch dressing mix – Almond butter – Coconut flour – Unsweetened cocoa powder

	– Protein powder
	– Coconut oil
	– Olive oil
	– Cooking oil (such as canola or vegetable oil)
7. Others	– Pie crust (for Leek Quiche)
	– Pepperoni slices
	– Buffalo sauce
	– Nuts (almonds, pecans) for energy balls and crisp
	– Unsweetened coconut flakes
	– Chia seeds
	– Peanut butter
	– Chocolate chips (sugar-free)
	– Gelatin (for Low-Carb Cheesecake)
	– Almond extract (for Low-Carb Berry Crisp)
	– Vanilla extract (for desserts)

Make sure to adjust the quantities based on the number of servings needed and personal preferences. Also, consider any additional items you may need for beverages or other snacks not included in the listed recipes.

Strategies for staying motivated on the Atkins diet

Staying motivated is crucial on the Atkins Diet because it's a lifestyle change rather than a quick fix. It requires consistent effort and discipline to adhere to the low-carb, high-fat dietary guidelines. Maintaining motivation ensures that you stay on track, achieve your weight loss goals, and transition into a healthier lifestyle. Here are Tips for Staying Motivated:

1. Establish a Routine to Celebrate Success: Establishing a routine to celebrate your success is a great way to stay motivated. This could involve weighing yourself or measuring yourself regularly. When you start to see how far you've come, it'll be easier to stay motivated. Celebrating small accomplishments can also be a great motivator. When you make progress, reward yourself however you like—with a massage, a long bubble bath, or a haircut that will make you feel great.

2. Drink enough water: On the Atkins diet, it is important to drink enough water. Eight cups a day is the standard recommendation, but the bigger and more active you are, the more you need. As long as your urine is clear or very pale, you are drinking enough. Sometimes your body confuses thirst with hunger. Staying hydrated can help avoid this confusion and keep you on track.

3. Eat regularly and include protein in every meal: Eating regularly and including protein in every meal is another important strategy for staying motivated on the Atkins diet. Whatever your stage, eat three regular meals and two snacks each day.

If you want, you can also eat four or five small meals throughout the day. Eating every few hours will maintain your blood sugar and energy levels and keep your appetite in check. Make sure to consume 4 to 6 ounces of protein for breakfast, lunch, and dinner. Taller men can have up to 8 ounces.

4. Finding and Eliminating "Hidden" Carbs: Finally, finding and eliminating "hidden" carbs in sauces, beverages, and processed foods can help you stay on track. These hidden carbs can add up and interfere with your progress on the Atkins diet. By being vigilant about reading food labels and understanding where hidden carbs might be lurking, you can avoid these pitfalls and stay on track with your Atkins diet plan.

Dealing with Plateaus

In the context of weight loss and dieting, a plateau refers to a period where you stop losing weight despite continuing with your diet and exercise regimen. This is a common occurrence for everyone who tries to lose weight.

During the initial phase of weight loss, you may experience a rapid drop in weight. This is because when you cut calories, the body gets needed energy by releasing its stores of glycogen, a type of carbohydrate found in the muscles and liver. Glycogen is partly made up of water. So when glycogen is burned for energy, water is released, resulting in weight loss that is mostly water.

But when you lose weight, you lose some muscle along with fat. Muscles help maintain the rate at which you burn calories (metabolism). So when you lose weight, your metabolism slows down, causing you to burn fewer calories than if you were heavier. Your slower metabolism slows down your weight loss, even if you eat the same number of calories that helped you lose weight.

To lose more weight, you need to increase your physical activity or reduce the number of calories you consume. Using the same approach that worked the first time may help you maintain your weight loss, but it will not result in further weight loss.

Strategies for dealing with weight loss plateaus

1. Watch for Carb Creep: 'Carb creep' refers to the gradual, often unnoticed increase in carbohydrates that can occur when following a low-carb diet like Atkins. This can happen when you stop counting carbs and start estimating your daily intake. It's important to be honest with yourself about your daily carb intake. Pull out your journal, and get back into the habit of writing everything down so you have a realistic idea of what you are actually eating. This can help you identify any 'carb creep' and get your diet back on track.

2. Decrease Your Daily Intake of Net Carbs by 10 Grams: If you have progressed beyond phase one of the Atkins diet, you may need to decrease your daily intake of net carbs by 10 grams.

You may have exceeded your carbohydrate tolerance while losing weight, and you may have exceeded your tolerance limit to maintain your current weight. Once your weight loss resumes, you can add your carbs back in 5-gram increments.

3. Increase Your Fluid Intake: Increasing your fluid intake is another strategy that can help you work through a plateau. It is recommended to drink at least eight 8-ounce glasses of water per day. Staying hydrated can help curb your hunger and is good for your skin and overall well-being.

4. Increase your activity level: Increasing your activity level can also help you overcome a plateau. Practice can help you reach a certain point. If you increase the intensity of your exercises, you may find that the pounds start to come off again.

5. Find and Eliminate "Hidden" Carbs: Finally, finding and eliminating "hidden" carbs in sauces, beverages, and processed foods can help you break through a plateau. These hidden carbs can add up and interfere with your progress on the Atkins diet. By being vigilant about reading food labels and understanding where hidden carbs might be lurking, you can avoid these pitfalls and stay on track with your Atkins diet plan.

Transitioning from Weight Loss to Weight Maintenance

1. Transition to a Permanent Way of Eating: Phase 4 of the Atkins diet, also known as the Lifetime Maintenance phase, is about transitioning to a permanent way of eating. This phase is not so much a phase as it is a continuing healthy lifestyle. The foods you eat in this phase are generally the same ones you've already been eating, but there are some foods you unsuccessfully tried to reintroduce earlier that you can now handle. You can still experiment with these foods as long as you stay close to your goal weight.

2. Continue Adding Certain Ingredients to Your Diet: In this phase, you should continue adding ingredients like full-fat yogurt, fruits, and whole grains to your diet. Finding more foods you enjoy will help you maintain a healthy weight without getting bored with your eating habits.

3. Equip yourself with the Knowledge to Stay in Control of Your Weight: The goal of this phase is to equip you with the knowledge to stay in control of your weight. This could mean continuing your Phase 3 lifestyle, or it might include adjusting your carb intake if your tolerance changes or you regain a few pounds.

4. Adjusting Your Carb Intake: If you stop losing weight or start to regain weight, you may need to adjust your carb intake. This could mean decreasing your daily intake of net carbs by 10 grams. You can then gradually increase your carb intake in 5-gram increments until you find the level that allows you to maintain your weight.

Remember, the ultimate goal of the Atkins diet is to move through each phase, culminating with the lifelong maintenance phase, which should become your permanent diet.

Moving from one phase to another will help you achieve and maintain a healthful weight, develop good eating habits, feel good, and decrease risk factors for chronic diseases such as heart disease, hypertension, and diabetes

Conclusion

As we draw the final curtain on the Atkins Diet Cookbook, it is with a sense of accomplishment and empowerment that we reflect on the transformative journey you've embarked upon. Your commitment to health and vitality has led you through the corridors of a scientifically-backed dietary approach that not only transcends fads but stands as a testament to enduring success.

The pages of this cookbook have not merely unfolded recipes; they have guided you through a culinary voyage with purpose. Each meal plan, every delectable recipe, and the carefully curated selection of foods have been crafted to align seamlessly with the principles of the Atkins Diet. As you savored the rich flavors of a Grilled Lemon Herb Chicken or relished the simplicity of a Keto Sausage Egg Cup, you were not just nourishing your body; you were making a conscious choice for lasting well-being.

Beyond the tantalizing array of dishes, this cookbook has been your compass in navigating the nuances of the Atkins lifestyle. From the inception of your journey, understanding the profound history and principles of the Atkins Diet laid a solid foundation. The benefits— beyond weight loss—such as improved blood sugar control and enhanced cardiovascular health, unfolded like chapters in a well-crafted story of health and vitality.

Delving into the science behind the Atkins Diet allowed you to grasp the intricacies of your body's metabolic symphony. The notion of ketosis, where the body transitions to burning fat for energy, became not just a concept but a dynamic force guiding your dietary choices. Each phase of the Atkins Diet unfolded logically, providing you with a roadmap for progressive weight loss and sustainable lifestyle changes.

Navigating the culinary landscape, you learned to discern between foods to embrace and those to avoid. The cookbook became your trusted companion, helping you stock your kitchen, plan meals, and execute recipes with finesse. Through detailed meal plans and a diverse repertoire of recipes, you discovered that a low-carb, high-protein diet need not compromise on taste or variety. It's a celebration of flavor and nourishment in every bite.

The Atkins journey extended beyond the plate, encompassing lifestyle choices that fortify your commitment to well-being. Strategies for dining out and handling social situations empowered you to make mindful choices in any setting. Incorporating exercise into your routine became a natural progression, creating a holistic approach to health that intertwines diet and physical activity.

As you traversed the path of the Atkins lifestyle, the cookbook equipped you with tools to navigate challenges and celebrate triumphs. Staying motivated, overcoming plateaus, and transitioning from weight loss to maintenance were not just theoretical concepts but practical guidelines woven into the fabric of your daily life.

This cookbook didn't just offer recipes; it empowered you with resources. Shopping lists simplified your grocery trips, and food diary templates became your ally in tracking progress. The journey wasn't solitary; it was a shared expedition where every tip, every piece of advice, resonated with the collective wisdom of those who've embraced the Atkins lifestyle.

As you stand at the conclusion of this culinary and wellness odyssey, envision a future where vibrant health is not a fleeting goal but a constant companion. The Atkins Diet Cookbook has laid the groundwork for a sustainable lifestyle—one where the choices you make today echo in the vitality you experience tomorrow.

In closing, this is not just the end of a cookbook; it's a continuation of your journey towards radiant health. Every recipe you've tried, every piece of advice you've absorbed, is a step towards a more vibrant version of yourself. Here's to embracing the extraordinary potential that lies within you and to the countless delicious and healthful meals yet to be savored on your path to a life of vitality and abundance.

Congratulations on successfully completing your Atkins Diet journey! We trust you found exploring the pages of this cookbook both informative and enjoyable. As you continue on your path to health and vitality, this comprehensive food diary serves as a strategic companion. It's meticulously designed to assist you in tracking your progress, monitoring your food intake, and gaining valuable insights into your dietary habits. Feel empowered to customize this template to suit your preferences or unique dietary requirements. Additionally, consider printing multiple copies of this diary to utilize for each day of the week. Here's to continued success on your wellness journey!

How to Use the Diary

Getting Started:

Before you dive into using your food diary, take a moment to familiarize yourself with its layout and structure. You'll notice sections dedicated to recording your daily meals, snacks, and beverages, as well as spaces for tracking your water intake and physical activity. Take a deep breath and approach this process with curiosity and commitment to self-discovery.

Recording Your Meals:

Each day, take the time to diligently record everything you consume, from your morning coffee to your evening snack. Be as detailed as possible, noting portion sizes and ingredients used in your meals. This level of specificity will provide valuable insights into your carbohydrate intake and adherence to the Atkins Diet principles.

Tracking Your Progress:

In addition to recording your meals, use your food diary to track your progress towards your health and wellness goals. Take note of any changes in your energy levels, mood, or physical well-being as you embark on your Atkins journey.

understanding of how the Atkins Diet is impacting your overall health and vitality.

Reflecting on Your Choices:

At the end of each day, take a moment to reflect on your dietary choices and behaviors. Did you stay true to the Atkins principles, or did you find yourself veering off course? What challenges did you encounter, and how did you overcome them? By reflecting on your experiences, you'll gain valuable insights into your habits and behaviors, empowering you to make informed choices moving forward.

Setting Goals and Celebrating Successes:

Use your food diary as a platform for setting goals and celebrating successes along the way. Whether it's reaching a milestone in your weight loss journey or mastering a new Atkins-friendly recipe, take the time to acknowledge your achievements and celebrate your progress. By setting realistic goals and tracking your successes, you'll stay motivated and inspired to continue on your path to health and vitality.

Daily Goals:

- Carbohydrate Intake:___________ grams

- Water Consumption: ___________ ounces

- Physical Activity: ___________ minutes

Breakfast:

- Meal:

    - ♥ Time: ____________________

    - ♥ Description: ____

    - ♥ Ingredients: ____

    - ♥ Portion Size: ___________________

- Carbohydrate Count: ___________ grams

Snack:

- Meal:

    - ♥ Time: ____________________

    - ♥ Description: ____

* ♥ Ingredients: ____

    * ♥ Portion Size: ______________________

* Carbohydrate Count: __________ grams

Lunch:

* Meal:

    * ♥ Time: ____________________

    * ♥ Description: ____

    * ♥ Ingredients: ____

    * ♥ Portion Size: ____________________

* Carbohydrate Count: __________ grams

Snack:

* Meal:

    * ♥ Time: ____________________

    * ♥ Description: ____

    * ♥ Ingredients: ____

    * ♥ Portion Size: ____________________

* Carbohydrate Count: __________ grams

Dinner:

- Meal:

    - ♥ Time: ____________________

    - ♥ Description: ____

    - ♥ Ingredients: ____

    - ♥ Portion Size: ____________________

- Carbohydrate Count: __________ grams

Snack:

- Meal:

    - ♥ Time: ____________________

    - ♥ Description: ____

    - ♥ Ingredients: ____

    - ♥ Portion Size: ____________________

- Carbohydrate Count: __________ grams

Beverages:

- Water: __________ ounces

- Other Beverages: ____

Physical Activity:

Type of Activity: ____

Duration: ___________ minutes

Reflections:

Challenges Faced: ____

Successes Celebrated: ____

Thoughts and Feelings: ____

Notes:

Recipes